Foot Health Myths, Facts & Fables

Podiatry Reflections

David R Tollafield

Front cover image

Dessin, Jambes et Pieds (*leg and foot design*)
Claude-Henri Watelet (1718-1986)

Watelet was an amateur painter, a well-respected etcher, a writer on the arts and a connoisseur of gardens.

ISBN: 978-1-8384137-2-9

Busypencilcase Communications

Cover adapted and design

Petya Tsankova

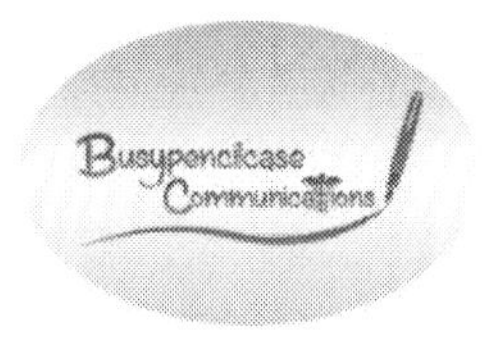

All photos are licensed through Shutterstock.com or from the author's library where patient permission was granted.

FOR READERS WHO SEEK OUT THE WONDERS OF THE FOOT

IN MEMORY OF LEWIS DURLACHER
(1792-1864)
A VICTORIAN PODIATRIST WHO
WROTE ONE OF THE FIRST FOOT
HEALTH BOOKS

Science can explain the truth only where scientific method is devoid of bias.

THE AUTHOR

Books by the same author

NON FICTION

Podiatrist on a Mission. The Genesis of a New Profession
(autobiographical-novel)

Promoting Foot Health as Podiatry*
Projecting Your Image. Conference to Village Halls (1)
PowerPoint is More than a Slide Program (2)
Bunion Hallux Valgus. Behind the Scenes.
Morton's Neuroma. Podiatrist Turned Patient: My Own Journey

With Linda Merriman

Clinical Skills in Treating the Foot
Assessment of the Lower Limb

*Replaces the previous edition Selling Foot Health as Podiatry

FICTION

Fatal Contracts
Shocking Short stories

The Story of Crystal Rouge
For children

Foreword

Professor Tim Kilmartin, PhD, FRCPodS
Ilkeston, England, & Hillsborough, N.Ireland

The first book ever written about the foot was by the French barber surgeon Rousselot in 1755 and described by Walter Selig two hundred years later. Unfortunately, Selig somewhat spoiled the back story. The title was *'Memoire sur les cors des pieds'* ('A Dissertation on the Corns of the Feet'). The book came about after Rousselot explained to his students that because he was so very, very clever, he could write a book about anything to do with the human body, even the lowest of the low: the foot. Even this might have been mythical in that he allegedly relied heavily on Daniel Turner's earlier book covering skin and such matters. Nicola-Laurent La Forest, surgeon-pedicurist to Louise XVI, published his own 'treatise' in 1781, (treatise being a name given to papers and dissertations before the 20th century). La Forest covered corns, warts, bunions, accidents of birth and deformities of the foot, which I suppose just about covers everything.

Royal connections seem to have been very important to these men, so I was delighted to see the author, who takes his place in a line of luminaries, references Lewis Durlacher, a surgeon-chiropodist to Queen Victoria around 1845. He also gave his name to Durlacher's corn. Although not quite Royal, Victoria and David Beckham also find themselves representing the footsore with their myriad foot problems. Although I have been a practising podiatric surgeon for well over 30 years, I found this book a delight. It is the case that the foot with its 19 muscles, 115 ligaments and 28 bones is unique. No other living creature has a foot that works quite so mystically and with such complex mechanics as that belonging to the human

Read this book, and you will find much about what it is to be human, not least the healthy dollops of sex and politics. But, unfortunately, in the 21st century, charlatanism in all its human forms is all around us.

This book will go a long way to dispelling some of the snake oil fantasies that can cost the footsore so dear. I found this book a very warm cocoon to lose myself in, and I was utterly absorbed and enthralled by it.

2021

Preface

Sometimes you can fix foot problems yourself, sometimes not. It would be good to keep away from all doctors or even podiatrists, but then sometimes you just have to seek out a qualified person because things get out of hand.

A massive marketplace drives health, and the foot health market is no less robust. The quest for information around health amongst the population of most educated countries is vast—most of what we read aims at providing information with advertisements.

The reason for a dedicated book on foot health, is because most books on simple foot health are written by non-foot specialists. *FACT* and *EVIDENCE* make for reliable reading. How does the reader navigate between good and bad advice, positive and negative, sales pitch and the genuine article?

We need to pick our way through those myths or fiction passed from generation to generation to arrive at the facts. It is best to know what is fixable without being taken in by mumbo jumbo ideas. There are plenty of books written by people who want to share their personal philosophy and charge a big buck. You cannot fix bunions with exercise or yoga -but you may feel better for relaxing!

Who should read this book?

Anyone and everyone with an interest in feet and foot health, but the content is aimed at the lay reader who wants more, but not as a full-blown textbook. This book is not a self-help book; however, it will help define self-help. In some sections I have delved more deeply than others. Most references today are accessible from the internet, and so you will see links. This is easier with a electronic book than paperback of course.

The would-be student seeking a career in podiatry could gain much insight as the scope of this speciality expands – the profession called podiatry blossomed from 1988 onwards from older roots – called chiropody.

Medical doctors often have little insight into the foot early in their careers. For the most part this distant ground level organ is relegated to the bottom drawer. Perhaps even this little book might appeal to them!

The substance in brief

The content primarily defines the causes of common foot conditions, without suggesting that you should have a go or what treatment is best. However, this is a treatise, to use the older name for a book, intended to demystify heavy science and remove prejudices.

Conditions are included that add to the image of the '*Ugh Factor'* which may appear familiar and even attract comedy; sweaty feet, chilblains, ingrown toenails and 'verrucas' - all too commonly thought of as disorders of no consequence.

Feet are an essential body organ. They are the first contact with the ground; the means to propel us forward, support us through our lives and allow us to climb, run and swim. They act as sensory organs that let us know what type of surface exists under our body.

This book is illustrated. Topics and questions are referenced and the content list will help locate subjects, together with the index at the end that can act as a cross-reference.

David R Tollafield
FRCPodS, MSc, BSc, DPodM, FRCPodM
September 2021

Content

What is anatomy?

- The bodily structure of a plant or an animal or of any of its parts.
- The science of the shape and structure of organisms and their parts.
- A treatise on anatomic science.
- Dissection of a plant or animal to study the structure, position, and interrelation of its various parts.
- A skeleton.
- The human body[1].

It has taken years for us to understand what lies under our skin. Those without such knowledge act blindly.

Anatomy is part of medical science applied to the human body. Before satnav and GPS, serious walkers needed to know how to read a map with all of its symbols and reference numbers - liken this to knowledge your clinician requires when it comes to anatomy.

Please use the picture on page 15 as a reference where bones and joints can be located.

Here is a general tip. If you want to talk about a joint just marry the two bones together where they connect. i.e talus and navicular becomes talo-navicular joint – '*simples!*'

---

[1] Freedictionary.com

Bones of the foot

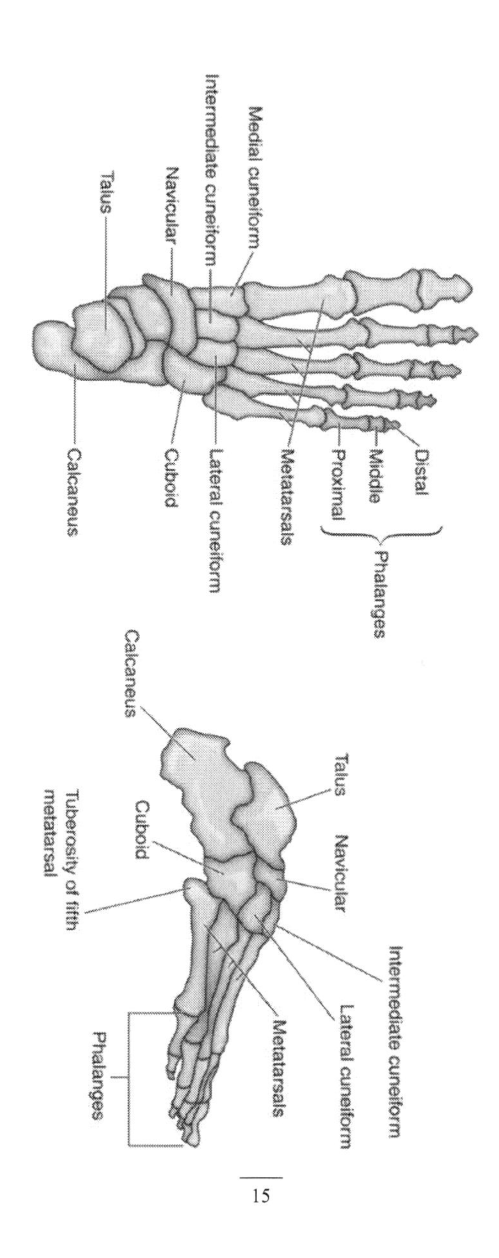

References

In order to simplify the source of the facts I have elected to use footnotes rather than ask you to turn to the back and find the reference. Please note that you may require a professional library to find the origins although some sources come from the internet where there is open access.

Abbreviations for the academic

The use of DOI, also known as digital objective identifier system is used and starts with 'doi' e.g

> Charkoudian,N. 2003 Skin blood flow in adult human thermoregulation: how it works, when it does not, and why May;78(5):6,03-12. doi: 10.4065/78.5.603

All internet or digitised references may not be accessible and hyperlinks are known to fail as work becomes redundant or altered in publications. This results in an error message appearing. As we edit and update our manuscripts, these problems do arise and so you are encouraged to let us know. To remind anyone not in the know, hyperlinks might appear as coloured text, or text that when clicked upon (selected) with the computer 'mouse' take you to a website or article. Tip – use the general title, author name (if given) and month/year in the search engine chosen if the link has expired.

In case you were wondering about the internet references - http stands for Hypertext Transfer Protocol Secure and is an extension of the Hypertext Transfer Protocol (HTTPS). Of course WWW stands for world wide web. Many searches do not require the prefix HTTP usually written as https://

1 - A bit of overview

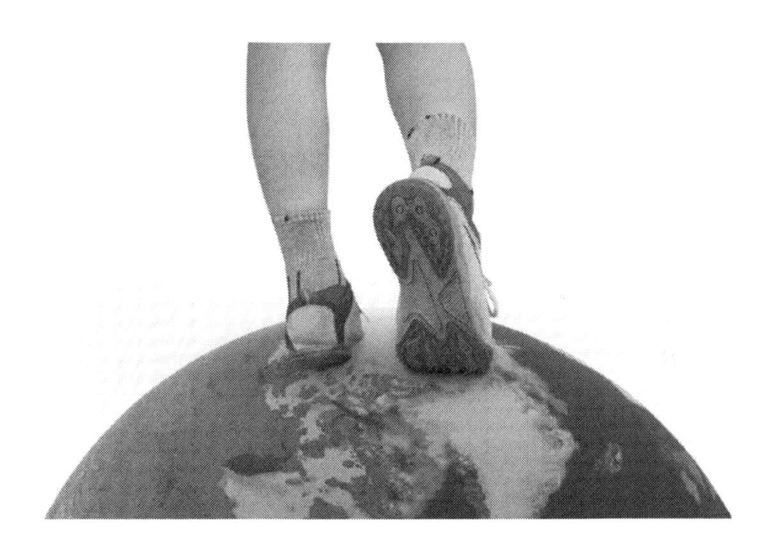

In the first chapter we will start with a little general information. Feet and ankles are as important to health as any organ in the body. A quick summary of the content is given on this and subsequent chapter pages.

- Common problems
- Poor Health
- Damaging the body
- Tissue recovery
- Fitness centres
- Previous injury
- Who deals with the foot?
- Pedicure – what is this?
- Foot and mouth!
- Do podiatrists help solve crime?

Fiction versus Fact

We all love stories, whether housewife tales or fables, like burying a piece of steak in the garden to get rid of warts, or preventing chilblains by keeping a horse's tooth in a pocket. Myths of course are tales or suggestions that in the end are not factual. Chapter 7 covers the concept of fables in more detail and holds out with a moral to the tale.

Do eighty per cent of peoplc have a foot complaint once in their life? And do we really walk 80,000 miles in a lifetime? Is this a tall tale?

Well, what about walking around the world in a lifetime - true or false? If we walk 10,000 steps a day, which can be a big ask for a westerner with a car, we walk around 3.31 miles per day. If we walk 80,000 miles, that comes to 1,142 miles per year, and provided we live to three score and ten, this could mean walking around the globe, three times, a distance of 24,900 miles.

Common problems with feet

The most frequent problems facing patients are ingrown toe nails, corns, hammer toes, bunions, neuroma (Morton's) and swellings such as ganglia – plural of a ganglion. These conditions, together with chilblains, nail fungi, heel bump pain and fasciitis (central heel & arch pain), represent the usual complaints seen by the family doctor or podiatrist. While surveys report these as key topics, when analysing data from my own website, a different picture emerges.

Foot bumps and lumps on top of the foot, heel pain, queries about the best age to treat bunions, what painkillers to use for feet and diagnosing foot pain. Then there are queries about why look after your feet and footwear?

Loss of sensation called peripheral neuropathy in feet, cancer, Covid-19 toes have emerged posing a need for awareness of signs that indicate clotting problems.

Questions

If we look at why people come to consult us and what questions they have, we have two different types of enquiry. Those that present face to face with clinics and those that seek broader questions.

Of course public articles drive the reader to the query in the first place and so in reality the queries people seek will only be recorded based on the meal they are served. Change the question and a different group of seekers will appear.

Is the article really what people desire? There are many questions perhaps not asked and so we need to present a menu of topics that prise open pandora's box. To a greater extent providing what a reader wants and needs is better than telling them what they should consider. Using an open forum seems the best way to find out those telling questions. The reader is also recommended to my website **www.consultingfootpain.co.uk** and other sources related to the foot and foot health.

Poor health

Patients in poor health are at greatest risk when it comes to feet. There are no myths in this case where problems associated with nerve damage (neuropathy) and diabetes occur. Some of these concerns are covered under the titles in this book such as shape, infection and skin. Perhaps we can look at damage and recovery as part of injury.

Damaging the body

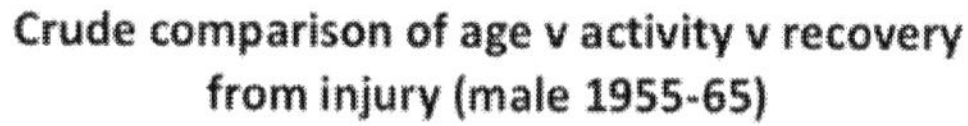

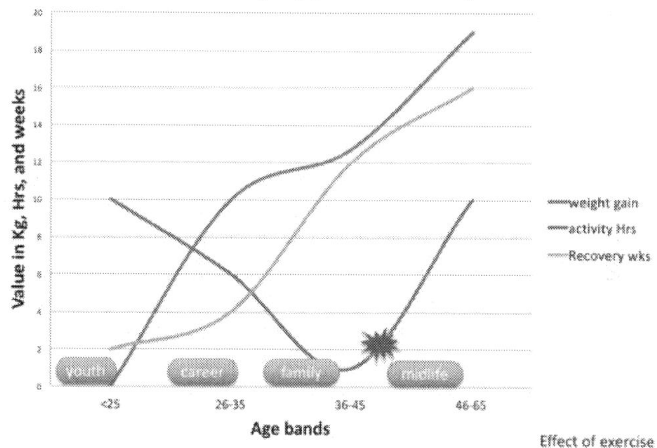

A case history

The graph above forms an interpretation of the timeline for age, weight gain, activity at work - before retirement.

The male subject in this graph was born between 1955-65. The bottom line follows ages grouped from under 25 to 45-65.

Youth, career, family and midlife are typical categories that impact on our activity. The starred explosion is the area when injury arose for this one case history.

The three lines relate to weight gain which rises as we age. Recovery following injury takes longer as we age and activity can reduce as we age.

Injury & Timeline

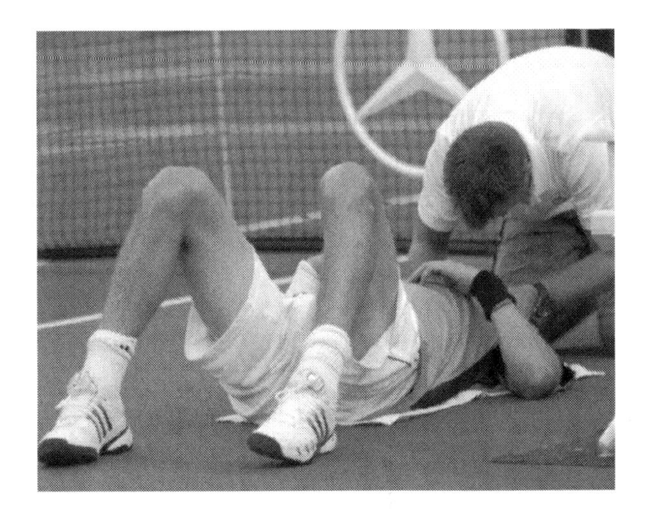

Injuries lie low for years. The visual graph used earlier expresses an assumed history based on the author's profile. Weight gain hits us around the mid-thirties to fifties. While our physical activities may start at school age and then follow into the next stage of life, exercise often diminishes when careers peak. Building a family home and a work career, often alters our attitude toward exercise until we reach a point where we don't feel so great about our body. This is a form of neglect. Admittedly some people do have a vigorous exercise ethic throughout their lives. A good colleague was a triathlete and Iron Man competitor. He still died before he was sixty from cancer!

Fitness centres

The promotion of fitness centres and our desire to lose weight has driven generations into fun runs. The message to stay healthy is essential.

However, people could still benefit from walking with tailoring exercise to their needs without subjecting their bodies to poor techniques from over straining.

Exercise is emphasised where a history of previous injury has arisen. It is not just feet, but all the structures of the musculoskeletal system – knees, hips, pelvis and lower spine that take the impact. Perhaps the message is not so much to keep running but use the expertise of professionals to design how we exercise based on the pre-existing condition of our bodies.

An assessment by a qualified fitness instructor would benefit before embarking on any ignorant use of a centre's exercise facilities. There is no myth - exercise is good for you, but poor use and knowledge can do more harm than good. Good quality fitness centres are an investment in health and recovery from injury.

Exercise will keep you living longer if you accept that you are better exercising modestly and eating well and enhancing your education in matters that sustain good health. There is no protection from early death but it helps if we believe we are better maintaining optimum health without injury.

Retirement & wellbeing

After retirement, and in some cases through mid-life crises for both males and females, the impact of early injury becomes more relevant. The graph cannot apply as a generalisation. Variables exist, but the graph does illustrate the effects of injury amplifying through life. Exercise and activity is good for us all. It is good for our body by supporting functional strength and feeling at one in our mind.

Those aforementioned tissues, tendons, ligaments and joints enjoy a little movement to remain in peak condition. Mental stress diminishes with exercise, helped by boosting our circulation which benefits our heart, lungs and brain. The corollary to this is that a wise man or woman knows when to stop if injured. Do you return to the very activity you once loved only to injure yourself again? The problem is how much recovery can we achieve after injury. Talking feet and ankles, well, this may vary. The effect on joints and tissues may allow recovery provided that the diagnosis was correct in the first place.

Optimum Treatment

Let's develop a scenario where you don't seek help, but your foot pain needs intervention years later. The treatment offered may work and allow you to continue your hobby or sport. On the other hand, treatment may be disappointing, and you believe the clinician you sought has failed. The variability in success following any medical management hinges on how much damage (pathology) was sustained, not just at the first injury but subsequent injuries. This is referred to as the *timeline*, which implies an optimal point in an injury cycle when the trauma to the tissues mentioned above will recover. Athletes are professionals and loss of their ability means revenue cannot be recouped during their recovery period.

The dancer

I interviewed Jenny, a former professional dancer. While Jenny never sustained a significant injury during her career, it was clear she had experienced chronic problems over the years. Her following comment perhaps underlies the pressure that professional dancers have to endure.

"I've probably had a lot of pain most of the time, and I think a lot of dancers do go through a lot of pain, but you just kind of get on with it. The worry of even mentioning it [pain] or anyone hearing about it because you don't want to tarnish yourself with an injury!"

The tennis player

The Scottish tennis player Andy Murray was in so much pain that he required his hip joint to be 'resurfaced'. Such restoration of the joint surface helped him recover, but his performance would suffer as he hit his mid-thirties as evidenced at Wimbledon 2021.

Seasoned athletes can cope with damage because they are psychologically programmed through years of training. Look at how managers now protect the highest paid footballers and select them for short periods on the pitch. Whereas when you or I would stand down, amateur and professionals continue. As a result of continued performance they will inevitably suffer from their injuries which, once acute, will become chronic.

We all age at different rates, but as a statement this is false because we all age. However, some look better than others at the same age. Pain ages us and affects us psychologically. It is worthy to note that we are not all designed to the same tolerances. Those who can cope best after injury do better if their mechanics are balanced to cope with the inevitable stress associated with exercise. Athletes perform at the top of their human ability.

Build a bridge out of insubstantial materials and it will collapse prematurely. Use an engineering design that can cope with the stress of movement in all weathers, and that structure will hold up and last longer. In some ways this is true of our human make up, and the framework about which we exist is called the musculoskeletal system.

Biomechanics and the human body

Biomechanics is a word implying the science of movement and forces applied to living tissues. The forces imposed upon normal tissue should allow it to deform and recover swiftly. MSK sciences emphasise how we deliver health around injury to joints and muscles.

Tissue recovery

Skin stretches and returns to its former shape as it is elastic. If hydrated it can cope with the daily stresses of life in shoes and bare feet. Cartilage deforms and restores its shape on movement within joints. Cartilage is soft and relies on a mattress of fibres interwoven with long chained molecules that trap water. In effect cartilage becomes stiff at the point of greatest pressure and softens to absorb that impact.

Tendons connect muscles to bone and are made of parallel fibres or strands of protein called collagen. Tendons have a lining which, like joints, is lubricated around the major parts of the body where tendons pull against bone. They have a pulley effect in many cases. The key pulley-like tendons act around the ankle and midfoot. Ligaments are flatter in general, have no contractile effect between muscles and bone and joints. They add to the strength around joints like guy ropes of a tent. Supporting the main skeletal frame is important by numerous ligaments. Bone must deal with forces and being made from collagen it also has a structure which absorbs calcium and phosphate to make it strong. Bone can withstand vertical, twisting and bending forces due to a combination of aero like bubbles inside (spongy) and a thick outer casing (hard). Each type of tissue mentioned copes with stress in different ways to support and protect the body.

Who deals with feet in the UK?

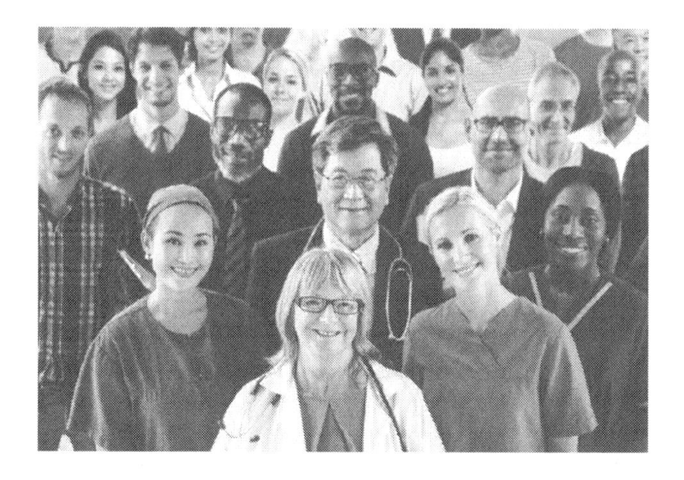

Podiatry is the only profession dedicated to total foot care health and management.

The Health and Care Professions Council (HCPC) was established in 2003 and covers most non-medically qualified professions. The HCPC was in fact a form of rebranding from a previous but similar regulator called the Council for Professions Supplementary to Medicine (CPSM).

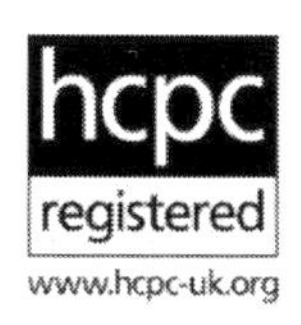

Physiotherapists and occupational therapists might be involved with elements of foot care and are HCPC registered. Osteopaths and chiropractors also manage joints and muscles and could be involved with assisting foot pain and regulate themselves but do not come under the HCPC.

Acupuncturists also deal with pain associated with the lower limb, but, regulation is less transparent.

Podiatrists overlap, they are HCPC registered and provide physiotherapy methods and in some cases, acupuncture and acupressure techniques as part of pain relief. Foot care assistants work alongside podiatrists. Foot Health Practitioners are qualified but do not have a national register as do podiatrists and do not form part of the NHS foot health service.

For more complex foot problems, patients can seek a podiatrist with extended training. These extended scope practitioners (ESPs) can help manage problems usually outside the care of the patient's general medical practitioner. Podiatric surgery came about from 1975 and now provides similar non-trauma surgery for a wide range of deformities at consultant level as in medicine.

Orthopaedic departments manage foot trauma within the NHS. Some orthopaedic surgeons overlap with podiatric surgeons for elective surgery. It takes around 16 years to become a medically qualified surgeon and 12-13 years to become a medically trained podiatric surgeon. Orthopaedic surgeons qualify as medical doctors first. Other surgeons specialise in vascular disease of the lower limb. While medical specialists cover rheumatology, cancer, skin diseases and endocrinology (hormones and metabolism), many clinical staff play a part in managing feet. The development of multi-disciplinary teams (MDTs) within both the independent and NHS sectors provide a wide range of care working together for the patient. The picture may appear confusing, but many consultations commence with the patient's general medical practitioner.

Mister or Doctor?

Anywhere else in the world, but not the UK, surgeons are called doctors.

In the UK, the surgeon is a Mister once they have gained their Fellowship. Fact! Surgeons gravitated from the industry of barbers and even tooth pullers. Anyone with a strong constitution could become a surgeon or saw bones. Physicians were better trained and regulated but by the 18th century some changes occurred that allowed the surgeon and physician to merge, but not on equal grounds. Surgeons played to an audience with floors covered in sawdust and tiered seats for viewers – hence the operating room is still called *the theatre* in the UK.

Is pedicure the same as chiropody?

Pedicure and manicure are similar in that they offer a cosmetic service for nails on the feet and hands, with some reducing hard skin. Formal chiropody no longer exists in the UK and has been superceded by the professional name podiatry in most English speaking countries. Training is different between the cosmetic side and the medical side of foot health management. Being *'medically qualified'* implies becoming a doctor of medicine. *'Medically trained'* gives reference to a healthcare professional adopting medical methods based around formal medical practice within their area of specialty. In the UK anyone can cut toe nails or buff up hard skin as this is considered what someone could undertake for themselves. Care homes for the elderly and handicapped can use care assistants to manage these tasks. Complex foot problems however should be managed with a professional person overseeing footcare. While the law can confuse, the titles podiatrist and chiropodist are protected. This means, if you use the term podiatrist or chiropodist without being registered to practice you are in effect breaking the law and can be prosecuted[2].

---

[2] Type in HCPC-UK.Com to locate the official UK website to find registered professionals. The register recognises fitness to practice.

Foot and mouth

A common joke we hear as podiatrists is do we deal with foot and mouth? F&M is a disease of animals but in humans, it is known as hand, foot and mouth. This something we don't deal with - so over to the medical doctor.

Two interesting facts about dentistry and podiatry

The first covers a copycat relating to dentistry. From the late seventies and early eighties a foreward looking podiatrist called Marcel Pooke (Northampton) helped engineer a change in how podiatry clinics looked. He pushed for a change from the old style clinic to adopt modern ergonomic electronic patient couches. Unlike dentistry, the specialty of podiatry is less well known and morphed from chiropody around 1988 onwards. Dentistry can be traced back well before the 19th century, but until the early 20th-century, chiropody was poorly formed. General practice now has more of a dental look than the steel fixed high chair. How times change, but who dismisses copying to improve?

The second fact that links dental health to feet surrounds the curious case of the ingrowing toe nail. We will meet this condition later on in more detail. When a patient presented with an infected toe, antibiotics failed to work until the culture sent to the laboratory came back with named bacteria specific to an oral infection. Maybe there is a relationship between foot and mouth afterall. Although rare, such infections are known as focal infections[3].

---

[3] From the authors own case notes. 'Prevotella species' arises from gingivitis or gum disease.

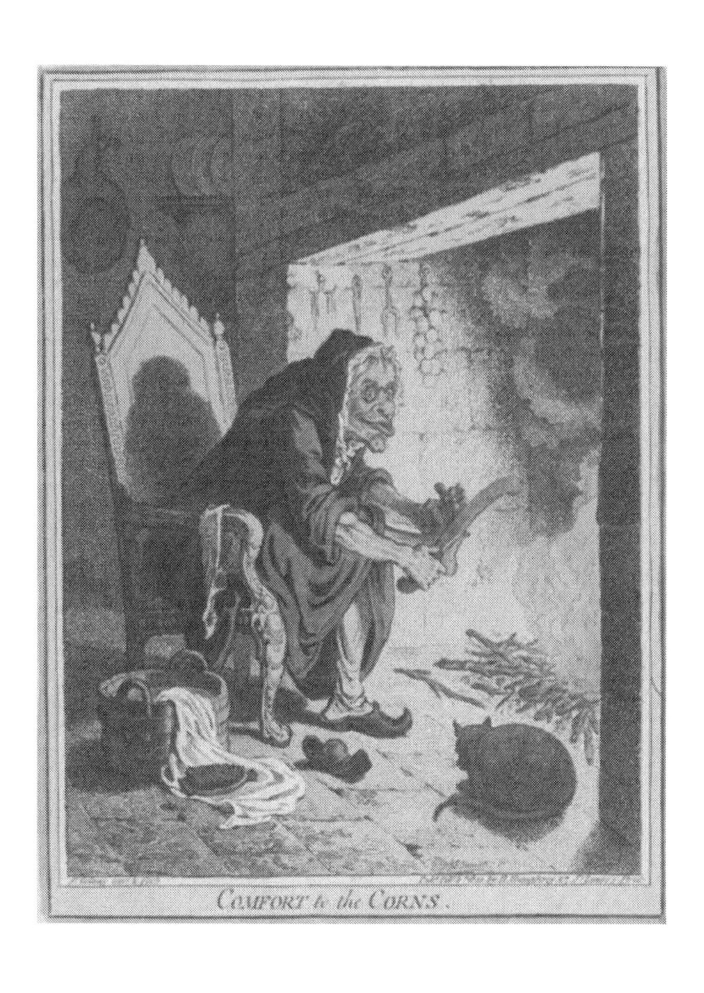

Illustration - James Gilray 1756-1815 *Comfort to the Corns* published 1800. Hand coloured etching on ivory wove paper. Published by Hannah Humphrey

Charlatans

We know that surgical chiropodists were recognised as far back as the mid-19th century because of various old publications. Early accounts and imprints, much as the cover of this book, suggest foot care management was popular in the coffee houses in cities. The well to do could afford this luxury but it did give rise to charlatans who pretended they could cure corns and would use fish scales to mislead their clients in justifying a visible cure.

A profession with a pedigree

After the eighties, degree courses led to a Bachelor of Science in Podiatry (BSc). Podiatric medicine is now the formal subject: three years in England, Wales, Northern Ireland, and four years in Scotland. Those podiatrists who qualified before 1988, and did not have a BSc, often retained their original title of chiropody alongside 'podiatrist'. The award DPodM was offered to signify that a formal course leading to registration had been completed. A small percentage of the original diplomates took a further degree or extended their original qualification.

In the sixties some chiropodists formed a sub-profession called podiatrists in order to practice surgery concerned that the foot had been relegated to poor orthopaedic practice. Today orthopaedic and podiatric practice is better regulated and performed with collaboration in many parts of the UK through multi-disciplinary teams.

Is there overlap between pedicure and podiatry?

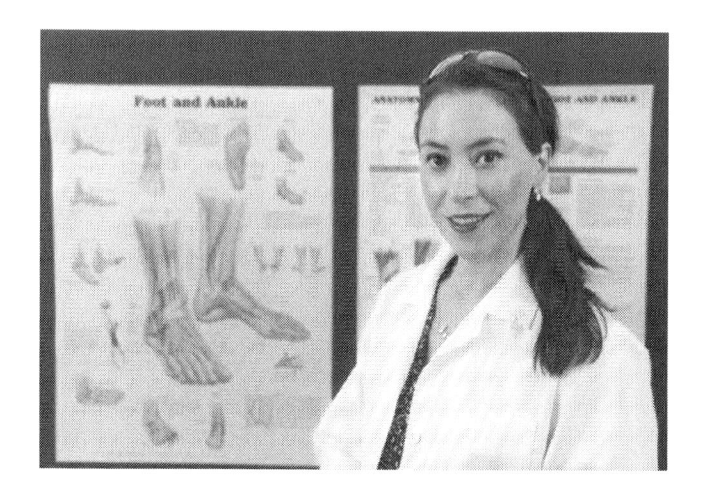

The only similarity between a cosmetic appointment and podiatry consultation is that skin and nail management is necessary to cut back nails and reduce bulky skin.

The modern podiatrist is required to establish a cause of pain and changes within the skin. The bulk reduction is often due to abnormal pressure across the foot, or skin infections and sometimes skin changes that require urgent management and diagnosis.

Nails and skin are exposed to cancer, although rarer in the foot than elsewhere. If podiatrists do not reduce the bulk of the cellular build-up, then damage beneath the skin and nails made from a protein will deteriorate causing pain, abscesses, and infection.

A podiatrist's training involves recognising common medical diseases affecting the foot and the lower limb. The profession provides a range of treatment, diagnostic skills and medications that pedicurists don't offer within their scope, as well as offering surgery.

Are podiatrists used to help solve crime?

The conviction of criminals depends on evidence. We have all heard about CSI (USA) and SOCO (UK)– Crime Scene investigator and Scene of Crime Officer. A small podiatric specialty has emerged over recent years, contributing a significant impact on a number of occasions within the criminal justice system. While the police will use their regular laboratories, podiatrists can assist police with patterns of walking, particular aspects of footwear analysis and footprints.

Podiatrists can apply their professional knowledge to help the police in forensic analysis and identification. A number of the cases have been high profile, and podiatrists' involvement has received coverage in the media and news programmes during Court proceedings and documentary programmes after the event where interesting cases piqued public interest[4].

[4] Additional information cited from advice provided by Professor Wesley Vernon OBE, PhD. Forensic Podiatrist. 29/7/21

There are postgraduate Master's degree courses available to those interested in pursuing this field of practice, and some forensic podiatrists work at PhD level to develop knowledge applicable to this work. Forensic podiatry covers four main areas – the use of podiatrists' knowledge in helping to identify persons from their clinical records, from bare footprints found at crime scenes, from their gait patterns (gait analysis) captured on CCTV cameras and finally from the wear and fitting features of worn footwear. Serious volume crime investigations benefit from this work.

Forensic podiatrists undertake defence work in criminal cases and, while not exactly always helping the police, such work can significantly assist the courts in their endeavours to seek the truth.

Media and publicity

Popularised by one police fiction writer, Peter James uses a real podiatrist, Haydn Kelly, in his Brighton based crime series. There are a small number of practitioners who work in this specialised area of practice and is known as forensic podiatry.

In terms of fictional portrayal forensic podiatry (FP) has also been included in BBC dramas (e.g. Five Days 2); CSI apparently bizarrely included a reference to 'there is an expert in Sheffield, England who can do this work for us'. Then there was one controversial episode of Bones (Canadian series about a forensic anthropologist based on the Kathy Reich's books) in which the main character was disparaging about a forensic podiatrist but then reluctantly, ultimately accepted that he had something useful to offer the world of forensic investigations.

Forensic podiatrist, Wesley Vernon, says -

> "The list goes on and apart from having advised the BBC script writer who wrote Five Days (season 2) I try to keep as far away from fictional portrayals of forensic podiatrists as I possibly can."

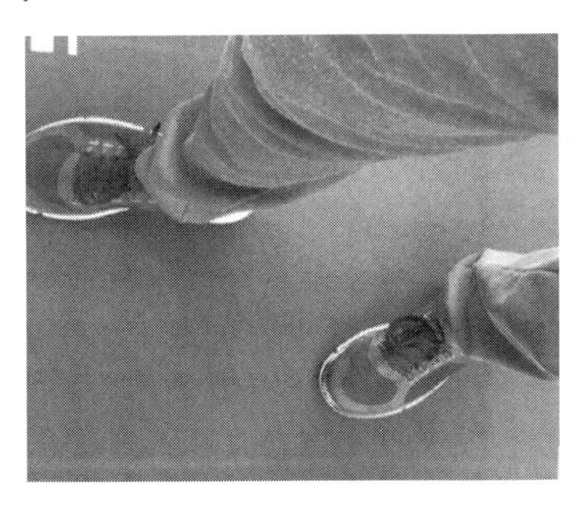

Gait analysis

Gait assessment means visualising a person's posture during movement, often on a treadmill of the variety seen in fitness centres. The way we walk is unique and can imprint on our joint movement. We limp or tilt in specific ways which includes our head, shoulder and arms - the latter arm swing may vary between people. The pelvis tilts differently between men and women. Injury adds to these changes creating that distinctive pattern. It is hard to change how we walk – so criminals beware.

2 – Skin

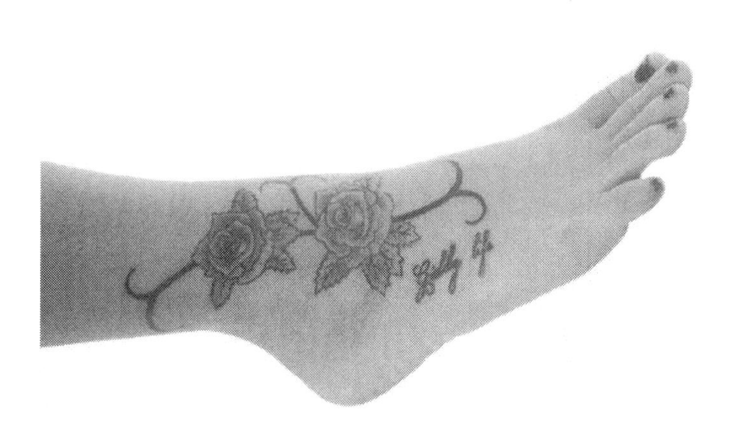

The study of skin comes under the medical specialism of dermatology. When it comes to feet, the skin appearance can change as a result of external influences, be it shoes, some type of frictional force or injury. The site of pain may be associated with adaptive changes such as hard skin to complex lesions – alterations to the structure of cells that are abnormal.

As a protector, the skin, made from the protein keratin, provides a barrier against infective organisms and maintains temperature control.

Colour changes give away the state of skin health and so redness is part of a sign that all might not be well. As the skin pigment darkens, racial and ethnic differences often become more difficult to diagnose. This fact has taken until 2020 to reach the foreground of medicine as most former published colour texts are shown with white skin.

From blisters to corns, sinuses and abscesses, small cuts and foreign bodies, we need to be alert to changes.

Skin forms such a large subject this chapter can only touch on some of the essential conditions we might attribute to myths.

- Trench foot
- Corny jokes and problems
- Callus versus callous.
- What happens to feet in space?
- Blisters and bursting
- Is it safe to tattoo my foot?

Corny jokes

Grandma's corns cause aching - true or false? Actually corns form over bone prominences but do occur due to injury to the skin. For some, they can tell the weather forecast and this appears to be the case when nerves serve as a barometer for the shift in air pressure. In actual fact this concept is more prevalent around amputation of toes. One friend had his fifth toe removed and could tell when the weather was about to change.

The sole of the foot, known as the epidermis, has the thickest layer of skin cells in the body. This makes sense as it is the first contact with the ground and we already know it is possible to burn through many miles in a lifetime (p.19).

When pressure builds up, the skin adapts forming callus which is different to corns. Corns are more seed like and this is how they acquired the name 'corn'.

Any podiatrist can tell you that when undertaking house calls, the pet dog seems to have an affinity for eating skin shavings following the process of layer reduction (debridement). There appears no rhyme or reason, but the same will go for nail chippings. The passion for keratin seems to attract them, but then we know dogs eat many things that humans would find disgusting!

A protein called keratin

It might be said that dogs eat skin and nails because of the protein, for that is what the essential structure is made from. Keratin is like a high class polish and repels everything from water to bugs which try to penetrate the body. It is a barrier. But what of nails as a weapon?

Would you argue with a rhinoceros? Doubtful, but those horns are made from keratin not ivory as in elephant tusks. Nails are functional on the hand but now of less use in feet.

Loose skin

Skin sheds its cells (squames) every 14-28 days depending upon your skin type and age and other factors associated with skin conditions. If you rub the skin below the ankle bones (malleoli) as an adult, you will feel a rough build up as you rub. The area of loose skin builds but disappears after a vigorous scrub. It is important therefore to rub vigorously to remove loose skin squames. In the disabled elderly, and those who cannot reach their feet, scaly reptilian like areas can make unpleasant viewing.

Do corn plasters work?

Podiatrists deal with corns and callus more than any other professional. The intractable plantar keratoma is the most painful kind of keratin-based lesion.

If the skin is hard and it needs softening, then keratolytic pastes are chosen as corn plasters. Keratolytics are chemicals that breakdown keratin; the -lytic part of the word, derived from lysis, means breaking down. A felt pad filled with salicylic acid (40%) paste will break down the corn, working on the cellular bonds called desmosomes.

Sharp blades

A scalpel in the right hands can reduce surface skin faster without the lengthy wait or risks of pastes which can cause unnecessary damage. However, not all corns are simple. Cross-sections through tissue from surgically removed corns often highlight inflammatory changes.

These types of corn are unlikely to clear because a) the changes are too chronic, and b) there is a pre-existing fixed toe deformity.

The sole can throw up even more concerns about what lies below the skin and makes clinical examination and diagnosis difficult. Hard skin with a crusty centre can be associated with organised sacs called cysts set deep in the tissue of the foot. The fallacy that surface management alone can provide effective treatment is misleading. Timpson[5] considered the effectiveness of debridement as being short-lived. In reality, most debridement is only effective between 2 days and one month. Dealing with complex skin problems in feet falls outside pedicure and a professional clinician with medical knowledge should be consulted.

Conclusion

Corn plasters can work by softening the bulk of skin that builds. The use of a scalpel is more effective. Corn plasters seldom do more than soften the surface. New established corns will benefit from corn plasters as long as the deeper tissue is not damaged or infected with viral tissue. Factual evidence suggests that long term use of plasters does yield benefit. However, corns are not just derived from the skin alone[6] and all the variables cannot be accounted when using this product[7].

---

[5] Timpson, S, Spooner, S K A comparison of the efficacy of scalpel debridement and insole therapy in relieving the pain of plantar callus. British Journal of Podiatry. 2005, 8(2):53-59

[6] Lopez, FM, Kilmartin, TE. Corn Cutting in the 21st Century. Podiatry Now. 2016.19(10):24-27

[7] Stephenson, J, Farndon, L, Concannon, M. Analysis of a trial assessing the long-term effectiveness of salicylic acid plasters compared with scalpel debridement in facilitating corn resolution in patients with multiple corns. J. Derm. 2016;43:6 https://doi-org.libaccess.hud.ac.uk/10.1111/1346-8138.13203

Callus or callous?

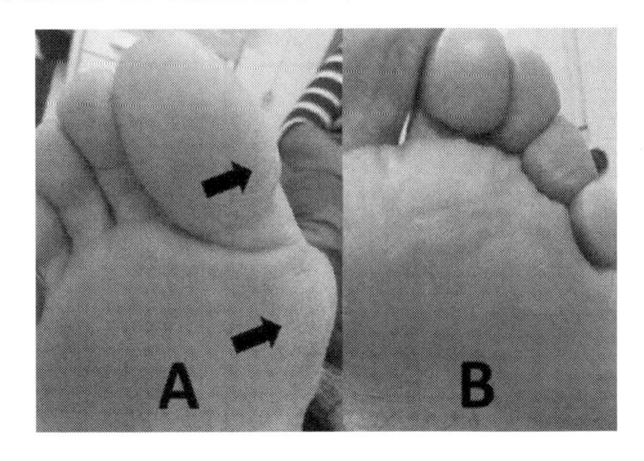

Callus is a noun meaning a localised thickening of the skin, and a verb meaning to form a localised thickening of the skin. Callous is closely related to callus, but it's figurative—that is, it doesn't describe actual skin—and it is never a noun. as an adjective, it means toughened or unfeeling. As a verb, it means to make or become callous[8].

So we now know we should use callus for hard skin. But should we cut callus? To make life simple I will describe two types of callus. (A) *physiological callus* that develops with exercise and foot position and (B) *pathological callus*, meaning that the skin and deeper layers have become faulty. Cutting down the bulk relieves pain. Ideally trimming callus to reduce this bulk can be conducted but it is better to try to find a reason why both arise. In many cases, the group in A will disappear if pressure is removed, deformity is corrected or an activity ceases. There is no evidence that cutting callus makes it grow as the layer from which skin cells develop is based on a pressure feedback system. Why not remove all pressure? Let's fly into space maybe?

[8] https://grammarist.com/usage/callous-callus/

Do calluses disappear in space?

The best way to relieve callus and pressure would be to achieve zero gravity. To put this theory to the test I found Scott Kelly and Don Pettit's blog which seemed to be evidential with a surprise twist. Scott and Don had been in space for 300 and 365 days respectively. Their blogs recorded interesting experiences. Because astronauts are not walking around on the ground under the force of gravity they don't have to wear shoes in space.

"The calluses on your feet in space will eventually fall off so, the bottoms of your feet become very soft like newborn baby feet. But the top of my feet develop rough alligator skin because I use the top of my feet to get around here on space station when using foot rails." Kelly

"After about two months in orbit your feet molt, and like some reptilian creature the callused skin on the bottom of your foot sheds, leaving soft pink flesh in its place, in the weightless environment, calluses apparently have no use, at least on the bottoms of your feet. However, the tops of your feet become red-rubbed raw and gnarly. And the bottom calluses shed faster than the top calluses can grow. Perpetually raw and hypersensitive, your foot tops can use a bit of padding to ease the pain." Pettit.

Pettit found the perfect antidote having grabbed a pair of small women's socks one day which protected the part that needed it[9].

---

[9] https://www.businessinsider.com/scott-kelly-weirdest-thing-year-in-space-2016-2?r=US&IR=T

Knives and cutting out skin

There is no doubt that people have been reported using 'Stanley knives' as a method of removing callus. The question is can this be done safely? No matter what podiatrists advise, and while outlets sell sharp apparatus, then such instruments will be used, occasionally causing accidents.

There are two viewpoints:-

The first is never use anything sharp that will cut because it is easy to slip. Remember advertisements are designed to make self-treatment look easy. Many people find techniques that can be copied are not always as simple to execute in practise.

It is no myth that knives are dangerous as we all know how easy it is to sustain a nasty injury in the kitchen. The engraving on page 31 is enough to make one shudder.

Feet are notoriously difficult to reach and even eyesight plays a factor. The second viewpoint is related to cleanliness. Blades should be sterilised after each use. Disposable blades are the industry standard.

Can abrasive modalities be used?

Simple skin that has little depth without complicated blemishes can be reduced with soft abrasive sponges, hand files or rotary drums. The cheese slice blades are equally dangerous although less so than open blades. It is better to stay safe and consult a clinician trained to manage feet.

If the skin is hard and has no difference in colour throughout, as long as circulation is sound, and the individual has no compromised health such as diabetes, then a rotary drum or abrasive sponge is a safe option.

Where the callus has different colours, think of a map of the sea seen from above with different hues of colour – green and blues – then do not attempt much more than surface reduction. Chronic callus is complicated and has different levels where small capillaries are easily damaged.

Are there nerves in corns?

Corns do not have nerves, neither do nerves grow into corns. Corns are made from the dense protein cells called keratin and have no blood supply. Therefore, corns are not vascular either. This misnomer is often taught at professional level. Remove a so called neuro-vascular corn all the way below the fat and put it under a powerful microscope and no nerves will be found. I have spent 40 years looking for evidence and have found none.

In 1845 surgeon chiropodist Lewis Durlacher[10] wrote about this phenomenon and for over 150 years the myth still lives on. The confusion arises because the deeper tissue often has foreign material or the skin may be infected by viral infection (warts) which cause the area to bleed and take on the sensation of nerve pain. The neuro-vascular corn perhaps could assume the name based on this complex appearance that deceives the clinician.

It is interesting to note that Durlacher who had some very wonderful ideas about treatment and defined corns thus: festered, vascular, soft and hard corns. It is interesting these older notations were replicated in my first year notes at University in 1975. A full depth excision of a corn together with underlying fat is shown over the page.

---

[10] Durlacher, L A Treatise on corns, bunions, the diseases of nails: and the general management of the feet. Simpkins, Marshall & Co pp 64-74

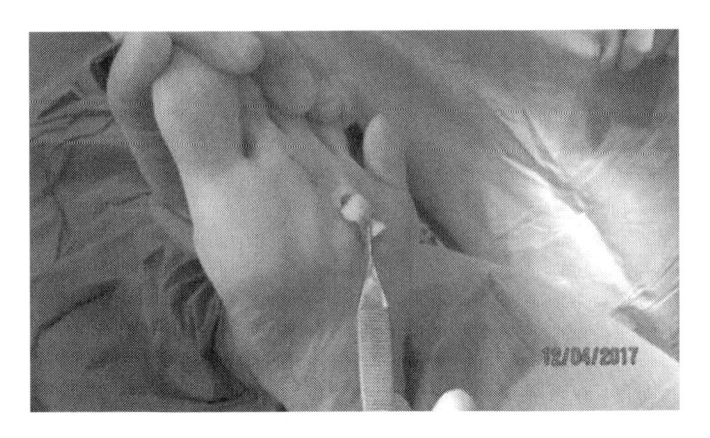

For the most part, our latter discussion concerns surgically removing corns. This is more relevant for the sole rather than the toes, where surgery is highly successful. If the corn is based around an infection, abscess, verruca or known dermatological lesion, then surgery plays a part. Freezing, heat - including microwave, are all fair approaches to effect a cure. Straight removal with closure of the skin can produce an unpredictable outcome by using a special skin flap (*Schrudde*) it is possible to gain some improvement by replacing the scarred tissue with new fat. Such actions should be used only as a last resort as success rates range from 40-70% on a conservative basis, although much pain can be eradicated even if the corn returns[11]. Long term follow up has never been presented.

---

[11] Saipoor, A, Maher, A, Hogg L. A retrospective audit of lesion excision and rotation skin flap for the treatment of intractable plantar keratosis. The Foot. 2018;34:23-27 https://www.sciencedirect.com/science/article/pii/S0958259217301232?via%3Dihub

Should you burst blisters?

As a rule, the raised surface of the skin should be left intact. In feet, blisters form due to friction from the skin rubbing, usually against a shoe. Excessive walking for long periods may cause the roof of a blister to burst adhering to the sock. The content is a thin liquid containing components of blood. These wounds should be cleaned, treated with a little antiseptic cream and dressed until healing starts to take place. As with any wound, treating early can avert infection.

If the roof of the blister remains intact the skin protects the wound from infection and should be left. A covering is a good idea to compress lightly over the blister but should not stick to the thinner skin because on removal the roof will rip away. The illustration shows a deroofed blister that needs covering while wet but should be left open when dry. Closed heeled shoes should be avoided if possible.

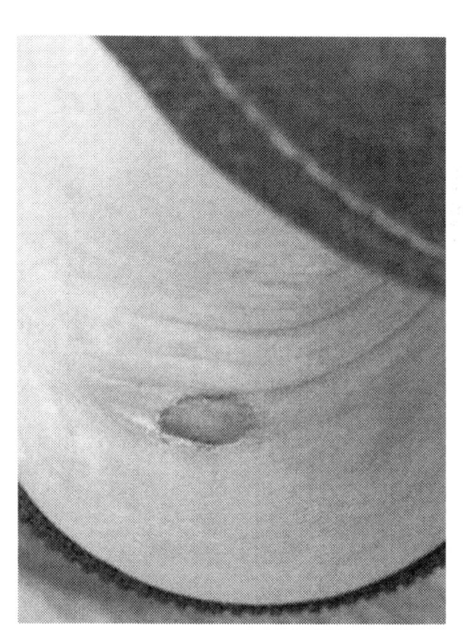

Is it safe to tattoo my foot?

Tattoos were once the mark of high society. That is a fact, tattoos have been around since before the 19th century. Tribal markings were important and most people will relate to those of the Maoris in New Zealand who carry spectacular images across their faces[12]. Today tattoos are popular and feet are no exception where the dyes or inks are injected under the skin.

Designs

There are two design approaches – the outline drawing or drawing with shading. The latter is more painful.

Depending upon the location of the tattoo on the foot, shoe rubbing can be uncomfortable, more so if an infection arises if the wound that forms is not kept clean. Tattooing is safe provided the artist is trained and adheres to the highest hygiene. *Tattoo Safe Register* exists in the UK which offers some level of assurance and their website offers more information on their role.

Tattoos are by design an injury to the skin. The ink potentially may react, as can any substance. Known allergies and sensitivities or poor skin quality and healing should attract *red flags*[13]. In other words don't have something done if there is a risk of a problem. Tattoos are painful especially when the area is large. Artists prefer larger designs to smaller designs. The top of the foot is pretty sensitive and exposed to more wear and tear over a tattoo. Protection of your tattoo is essential both after the acquisition and later on from sun and fading. Infections will certainly mean time off work.

---

[12] https://www.tattooswithmeaning.com/maori-tattoo-meaning/

[13] 'Red flags' are used in a wide range of protocols for warning signs

3 - Shape

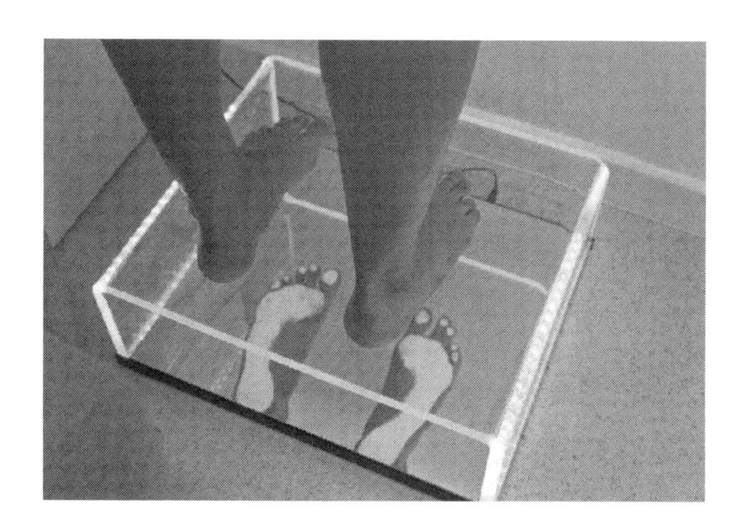

If skin is part of the common complaint associated with foot health, then bones, together with their joints are another major component that contribute to shape. How many face types are there? Google the question and you might find anywhere from five to seven types based around shape. When it comes to the foot we might suggest three shapes – but then that assumption is around normal. The arch is the target for our eye but there are more shapes than three because we have broad, narrow and a middle width in the forefoot. The hindfoot also can be broad and narrow. Add all of these together and it is no wonder why fitting shoes can be a problem. Let us have a look at some of those variations that step outside 'normal'.

- The steering wheel – talus
- Accessory bones – sesamoids
- Sexy toes
- Without toes!
- Exercises for toes
- The arch and the enemy
- Fascia and the foot
- The Orthosis
- Tailor's bunionnette
- Bunions – the big toe
- The ganglion

Foot Bones

The steering wheel

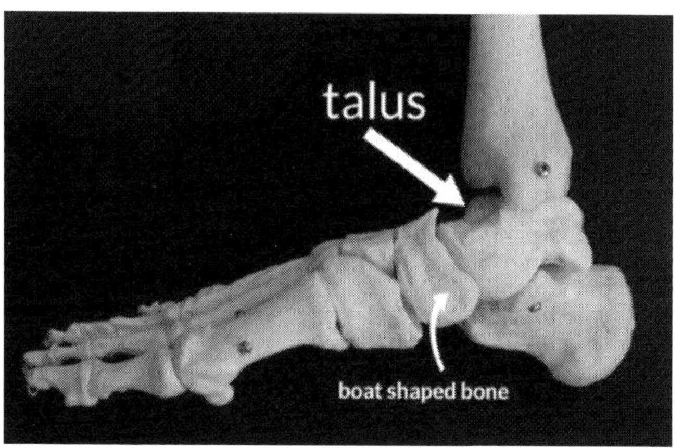

Maybe this is a little simplistic, but the foot moves on the bone called the TALUS. This bone can be found below the leg bones (tibia-fibula) and above the heel bone (calcaneus). This is the so-called foot's steering wheel. The name 'talus' comes from the Latin word that related to dice used in a Roman craps game and was taken originally from the horse as a convenient shape and size.

Modern dice are somewhat smaller of course, but the basic shape of this bone is rectangular and has a curved top surface. The talus faces the toe end of the foot and has a defined connecting dome that sits in a concave-shaped bone called the navicular or 'boat shape'. It is the closest design to the hip joint, except that it does not have the same broad range of movement. Shapes of bones around joints are essential for stability. Where the talus moves, or doesn't move, the remaining foot moves or doesn't move!

Feet are designed to walk without pain and should function over variable terrain; the ankle's design breaks down into three joints around the talus. The talus forms a connection between the hindfoot to the midfoot. A good deal of pain, plantar fasciitis and metatarsalgia, the generic name for pain under the ball of the foot, arises where the talus fails to stabilise the inside foot. The idea of the foot being flat emerges from problems around this bone and we will challenge the myths surrounding the flat foot later.

How many bones are in a foot?

Patients often say "*the foot is complex because there are so many bones*". The usual number of bones are 26 with 28 for two seed like bones called sesamoids. The fifth toe, like all of the toes has small bones called phalanges. As with all anatomical names these arise from the Roman language of Latin. Unlike the middle three toes, the little toe sometimes has two phalanges fused as one. The first toe consistently has two phalanges compared to the smaller toes with three bones.

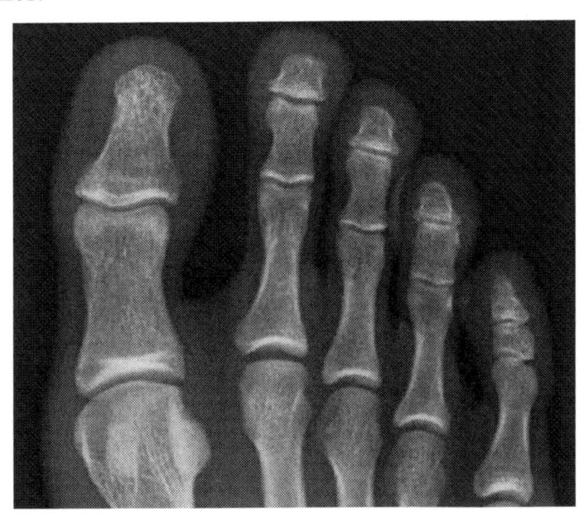

Accessory bones

There can be numerous accessory bones. These are add-ons but not counted as part of normal anatomy. Accessory bones are often silent and cause little trouble. However, and back to the subject of over exercise, some accessory bones spark off complaints. So, where are these bones? The percentages vary between populations and race. Of the consistent additional bones, sesamoids, number two, so 28 is correct.

The sesamoids of the first metatarsal are frequently overlooked when counting bones. They are not accessory but form part of a vital pulley system (see next image). Patients often look at x-rays and ask, *"what are those bones there, are they normal?"*

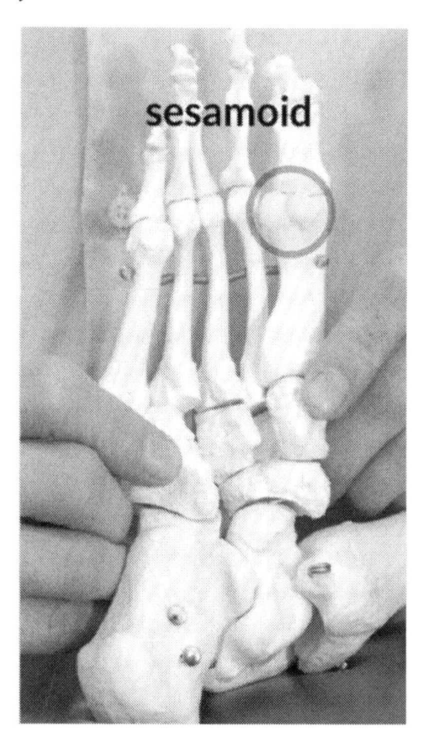

Can sesamoid bones hurt?

The surfaces of the metatarsal and sesamoid are sometimes rough and scrape together. Sesamoiditis suggests that the bone or the tissue around the bone can become inflamed, although the small muscle also adds to stiffening the big toe joint as it tightens with spasm. The largest sesamoid in the body is the knee cap, forming part of the knee's pulley system connecting the thigh muscle (quadriceps) and inserting below the leg bone (tibia). The knee cap or patella (p.76) enhances the efficiency of the knee. The first metatarsal sesamoids do the same thing.

The Os Trigonum provides an example of an accessory bone behind the ankle. The meaning of Os is bone, and trigone means triangular. Because the bone only exists in 7-14% of patients, it is different to the sesamoids, which are permanent features. The os trigonum exemplifies many accessory bones in the body. Injury traumatises these bones during stressed activities such as dancing and football.

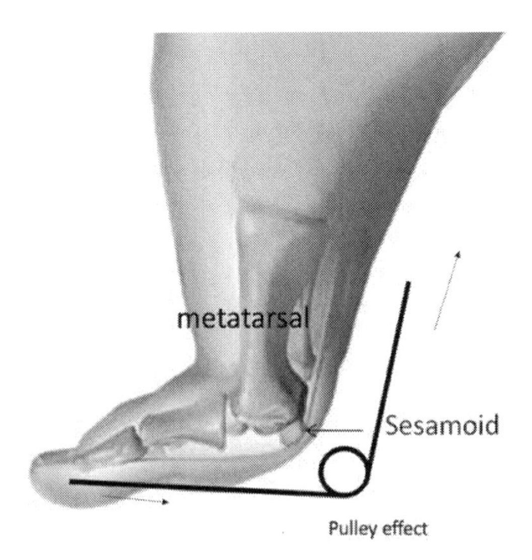

Why is the sesamoid bone called 'Luz'?[14]

After hearing that the sesamoid bone had a special spiritual name I decided to look further... In rabbinic Judaism—the relevance to the evolution of the concept of death—was that of the "bone called Luz or Lus". Luz means *almond tree* from the Hebrew and was associated with a Canaanite city. The bone was related to everlasting life. The 'bone called Lus' was considered important and held in high esteem as a mystic in religion. Given that this book is about myths, facts and fables, it is hard to resist a little more detail around bones, so forgive a little nonsense story ...

"Rabbi Ushaia AD 210 describes the bone of Luz in his book Bereschit Rabbi or Glossa Magna In Pentateuchium -great tongue of the five first books of the old testament –that there was a bone in the human body, just below the 18th vertebra that never dies. He suggested this bone was the repository of the soul after death; *IT* 'should never be burned or corrupted in all eternity for its substance is of celestial origin and watered with heavenly dew, wherewith God shall make the dead rise as with yeast in a mass of dough.' To add to the confusion, the bone of Luz might well have come from another part of the skeleton, such as the sacrum or coccyx, or elsewhere. The myth caught on, but the sesamoid was not a likely candidate.

The emperor Hadrian once asked Rabbi Joshua between the first and second centuries how God would resurrect people in the world to come. The Rabbi, a distinguished Rabbinic teacher, answered, *from the bone Luz in the spinal column*.
He had then produced a specimen of such a bone, which could not be softened in water or destroyed by fire. When struck with a hammer, the bone had remained intact while the anvil upon which it lay shattered. Vesalius showed that the bone did not exist in 1543."

[14] Lost Souls Helal, B The Great toe sesamoid bones: The Lus or Lost Souls of Ushaia. Clin. Orthopaedics & Related Research 1981 157;83-87

A Tale of Pain and the Sesamoid

The sesamoid bones are essential and serve as a lever to aid the great toe during that final push-off phase known as 'propulsion'. Ioosiffidis, an orthopaedic surgeon, wrote for 'Second Opinion'[15] about the condition of sesamoiditis. Bear in mind the -suffix of the word *-itis* means inflammation. His article is pithy and '*cocks-a-snook*' at politicians while indicating how medics can make decisions which lead to catastrophe. And so we have a sesamoid bone that is troublesome to a female and surgery is embarked upon. Conservative care was less than well-considered, meaning surgery was selected. The lady ended up with multiple surgery and, lastly, amputation of the foot. She developed a complex pain syndrome. The old proverb comes to mind and dates before Benjamin Franklin[16] wrote this in 1758; '*for want of a nail the shoe was lost...*'. The surgeon, however, used an updated version of the Scottish proverb from James Kelly (1721), '*He had need of a long Spoon that sups Kail [broth] with the Dee'l'*

The moral behind this tale and proverb highlight the need for caution in the face of a problem that might have been solved by simple means and yet undertaken by someone with knowledge and experience. Ironically this consideration was the basis upon which Hippocrates Oath was formed – *not to make the patient worse!* While all of this may mean little to the lay reader and novice, sesamoiditis remains a condition that still flays the best professionals. Sesamoid pain can be challenging to resolve. However, one has to be a brave surgeon to remove a foot for sesamoiditis.

---

[15] Ioosiffidis, A. If You Sup with the Devil. Second Opinion. Take a Long Handled Spoon. Clinical Orthopaedics. Pearson. 1995,9:61-69

[16] https://en.wikipedia.org/wiki/For_Want_of_a_Nail

Myths and facts about toes

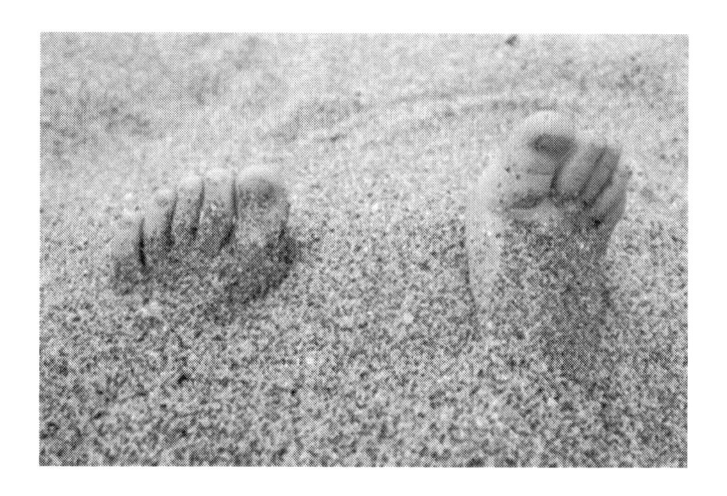

Are toes sexy?

This is a family book so I have to, forgive the pun, tread carefully. Toes are attractive to some and ugly to others. Nowhere are we more aware of the analogy that small feet are more beautiful in some cultures than others. The idea that a large foot is ugly is a fallacy and personal. Small people have large feet and larger, taller people may have proportionally smaller feet. It has been said all policemen have large feet. This might be true compared to the remaining population, but bear in mind the idea that all policeman have big feet is not true as a generalisation. Taller height and longer length legs have a trend for longer feet.

Is Communism good for feet?

The Chinese adopted the practice of foot binding. Several sources have been recorded in different eras. The idea to create a small Lotus foot was a symbol of beauty with the creation of a high arch. The toes and foot were compressed in bandages from a young age, impeding growth and forcing the foot to concertina into this supposed beautiful arch[17]. The origins of binding may have come from the fact that allegedly, King Zhou, the last emperor of the Shang, had a favourite concubine named Daji. She was born with clubfoot (below). This is a congenital condition seen infrequently and treated often within three months of birth in developed countries. The heel is small, the heel cord tight and the front of the foot twisted inwards. Left untreated the foot is smaller and has a higher arch.

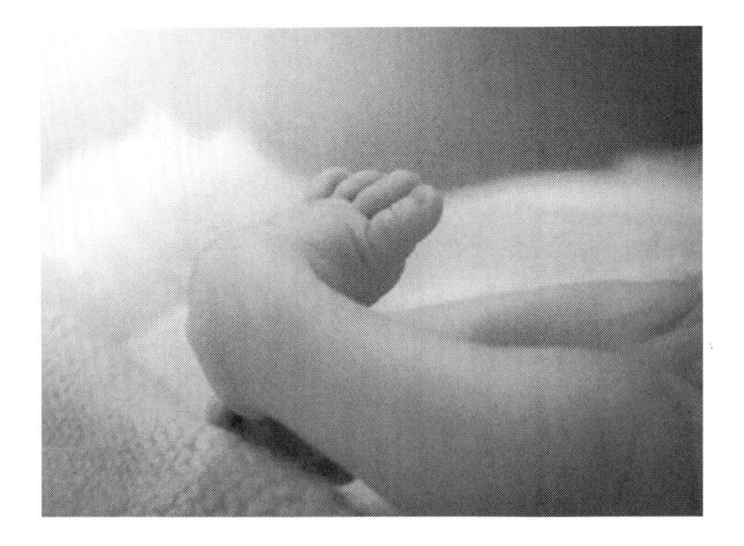

[17] Dutkiewicz Rebekah 2009 The Chinese Tradition of Foot Binding https://www.mtholyoke.edu/courses/rschwart/hatlas/mhc_widerworld/china/foot_binding.html

According to the legend[18], the sadistic Daji ordered court ladies to bind their daughters' feet so that they would be tiny and beautiful like her own. Daji was later executed, and the Shang Dynasty soon fell. Without a sponsor the practice of binding would not have continued and yet of course that is just what happened. In another tale, an Emperor called Li Yu had a concubine who performed a "lotus dance," similar to en pointe ballet. Because she bound her feet before dancing, she set a trend inspiring other courtesans and upper-class women to follow suit. Girls from six to eight years of age in society then followed this practice which was not outlawed until Missionaries visited China from the late 19th century. From 1911 the practice diminished and was outlawed with the Mao Zedong change in government in 1949 and the start of the Communist regime.

Can we live without toes?

The big toe does perform much of the work when we push off against the ground in a movement called the propulsive phase of gait. The foot twists a little and smooths out our forward progress when in contact with the ground. The remaining four toes also smooth out walking. They provide a spring to the step and offset the load (pressure) across the forefoot. Of course we can walk without toes, but will balance be affected? The answer will depend which toe(s) are involved. The natural bounce and shock absorption will change if all the toes fail to function. As with most problems some element of compensation occurs. Deformities and amputations are the main causes of reduced toe function.

---

[18] Szczepanski, Kallie. "The History of Foot Binding in China." ThoughtCo, Feb. 16, 2021, thoughtco.com/the-history-of-foot-binding-in-china-195228.

Why are toes named after tools?

Hammer and mallet toes get their name because the ends look bent down and adopt stiff joints. However these are not the worst toe deformities. Toes that are dislocated or retracted fail to touch the ground and perform no purposeful function. If anything this lack of performance increases the pressure under the foot causing pressure problems. The causes associated with deformities are mainly mechanical or medical disease e.g severe arthritis, but can be associated with poor fitting footwear and socks.

Reasons to amputate

Amputation surgery is a salvage treatment reserved for the dysfunctional digit offering faster healing with fewer problems than complex surgery. The decision to amputate a toe depends upon the patient's deteriorating health, lack of home support and social care. Such surgery can increase mobility and speed up healing from ulcers, infection and painful problems due to irretrievable deformity. Of most significance amputations offer rapid mobilisation offsetting problems from extended recuperation following surgery. The overriding risks imposed by maintaining unsuccessful conservative care allows surgery to become conservative.

Benefits of conservative surgery

Contrary to the tale of sesamoiditis, where surgery is employed, while there will be some loss of function without toes, the benefit from reducing pain and infection, with faster healing after surgery, outweighs most other considerations. The myth that you cannot cope without toes is false, but people can cope even without prosthetics.

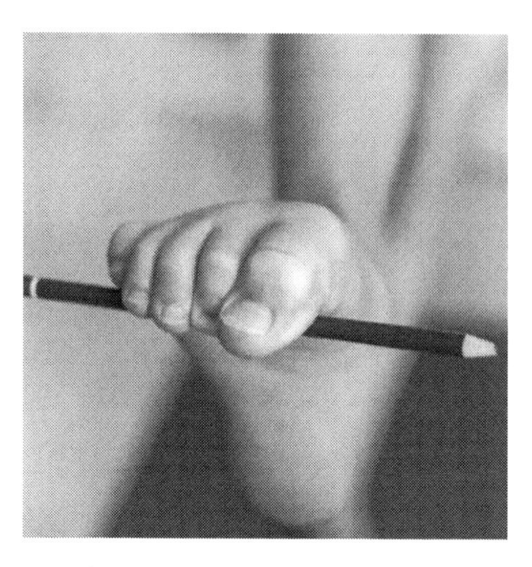

Do toe exercises prevent or help toe deformity?

I only have to read that picking up pencils with your toes will help, and I know the site probably stands as much chance of producing a rabbit from a hat as does an Easter egg producing a chick! However, it would be churlish to dispel the myth that pencils can help without some objective debate. Many years ago, the Distiller Company produced a drug to help with sickness in pregnancy. The net result affected congenital disabilities that caused limbs to fail to develop in the foetal stage. Those victims were able to use their feet and adapt to develop the same dexterity as with hands. For people without a need to convert toes to functional fingers, the benefit of picking up pencils or marbles would activate the flexor muscles. Here is what one site publishes,

In the next quotation (p62), there is no mention that the band of tissue called fascia ideally should be stretched as a profitable benefit of exercise. Picking up pencils works against this concept. In other words the quotation is poorly conceived and a different exercise should be implemented.

> "Foot-strengthening exercises promote long-term healing of plantar fasciitis by sharing the load of weight distribution and impact, as well as stabilising gait problems and pronation — both of which commonly cause or worsen plantar fasciitis."

Evidence for healing plantar fasciitis with pencil clutching is spurious. Where muscles in the feet function poorly, dedicated exercise on reaching adulthood is not easy, least of all benefitted by toes picking up objects.

Misdirection

Clever advertising can cause scaremongering with misleading language. The idea that exercises can achieve so much leaves mixed messages. Search engine returns, when making internet enquiries, may lead the reader down the wrong path. This is typical where subject matter you seek does not marry to the question asked.

By over activation of the toes in pick up mode, the movement is called flexion. The muscles and tendons worked are flexors. It just so happens that the flexor power in the foot outweighs the extensor power. As most toe deformities result in bending at the knuckle, undertaking excessive flexion accentuates the deformity. The weaker small muscles, previously called worm-like, are ineffective in overpowering the flexors even though they assist in keeping the toes straight. In contrast, with fingers, this is not a problem as the small muscles are well developed.

Check out your ability to spread the fingers wide. These are those same muscles in the feet that are weak because the toes are so much shorter.

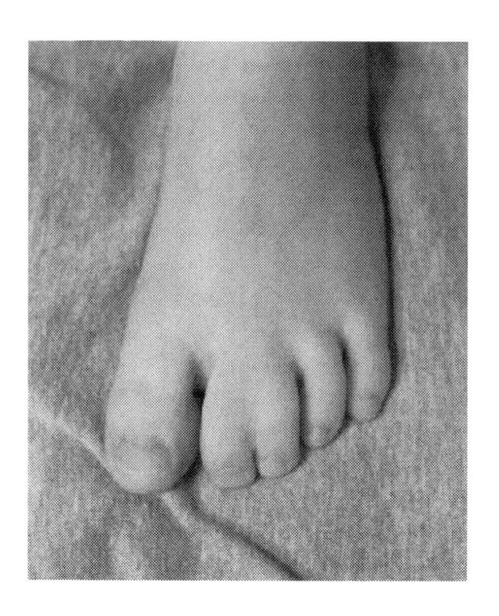

Do web toes help swimmers?

The image of humans with feet like flippers seems far-fetched but on rare occasions toes are joined together. This is called syndactly – joined toes. See the illustration above. It is far more common to have partially joined web spaces than full webs where there are no gaps. Now let's look at swimming.

The swimmer is trying to be torpedo shaped. Slim fitness means carrying no extra weight or fat. Too much fat means we will float more readily. Powerful shoulder muscles and legs propel the body. The feet play less of a role as motion comes from the hip. The presence of skin between the toes is irrelevant as are the toes. Once perhaps as important as fingers, toes have lost much of their functionality if we trace our origins back to apes and chimpanzees. I should add that the procedure of separating toes in order to restore a gap is not a good idea because the toe circulation is fragile.

Which is the closest animal to man?

Our foot structure and that of the chimpanzee is undeniably similar. There is one difference; the flexibility. This is brought about by the opposable digit like the thumb in the hand. But look at the mid part of the foot marked TT joint[19]. (B) human (C) chimpanzee.

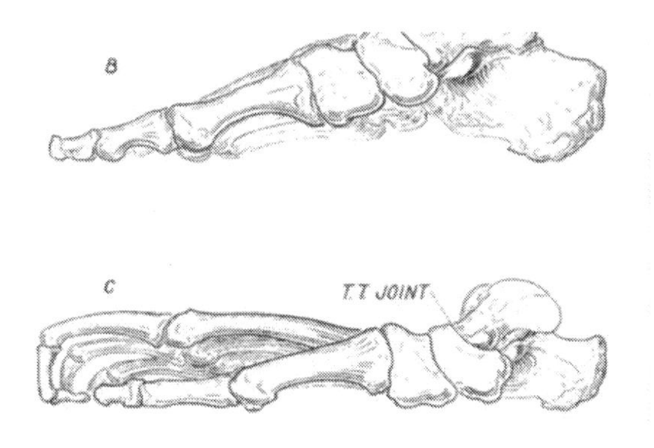

The heel bone in the chimp foot is smaller as it has not adapted to the human erect posture and heel toe walking style. Longer than toes provide more help with tree climbing.

---

[19] Schultz AH (1963) The relative lengths of the foot skeleton and its main parts in primates. Symp Zool Soc Lond 1963,1, 199–206.

Am I a witch if I have more than five toes?

You can have more than five toes and still not be burned alive or drowned. A sixth toe is called polydactyly or supernumerary and is found on both feet as a result a genetic predisposition. While uncommon, extra digits can arise from an extra metatarsal[20] or an extra toe bone (phalanx). The x-ray shown below illustrates a branched fifth metatarsal forming two complete digits. Purchasing a shoe with a wider width is required. This can cause problems if the back of the foot is narrow. Where psychological concerns arise, surgery can be performed to remove the extra digit. However, many patients live happily with a sixth toe.

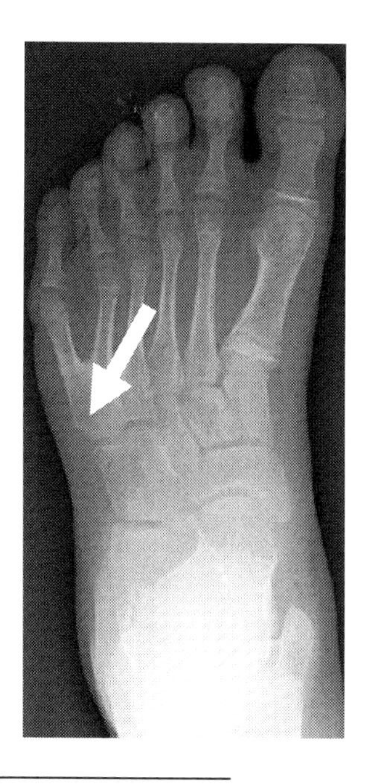

[20]https://upload.wikimedia.org/wikipedia/commons/d/d8/Polydactyly_01_Lfoot_AP.jpg

The Arch & the Enemy

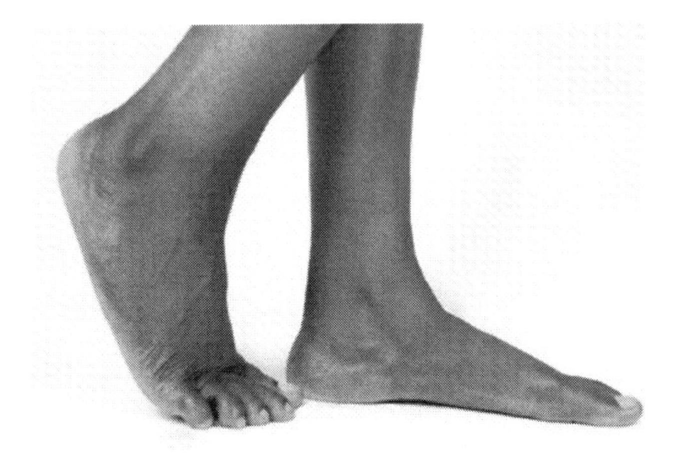

If the Chinese thought high arches were beautiful, then the low arch has been considered the opposite. *True or false?* We now move to a different story and one that begs the question...

Can we influence the arch with electricity?

One of the first ways to manage a flat foot was considered stimulation of the small muscles. Scientists from the eighteenth century such as Galvani in Italy (1791) had pioneered the advent of electricity used in animals.

The use of electricity to stimulate muscles became a significant development in medicine, not just for feet. The foot's small muscles cannot respond to any significant stimulus, and certainly not for the long arch. These muscles are 'worm-like' as one group is known - lumbricals (lumbricales). The other set of muscles, known as interossei, lie between the metatarsals.

The external leg muscles actually assist the arch shape.

How many 'arches' does a foot have?

The obsession with arches has led to a mega-industry issuing insoles and arch supports. *So do they do any good?*

During the first part of the 20th century in Britain, a flat foot excluded any foot soldier from the army, making the decision a travesty. Many athletes perform well with flat feet and yet an industry of speculators make spurious claims. *Is this a good sales pitch?*

There are three ideas about arches, and this is not to do with shape, but to do with where they are in the foot. The picture (p.70) shows the side view. This is a low arch foot, but the arch is the long or longitudinal arch. The second arch called the transverse arch which you will see likened to a humped back bridge. More about this soon, but the myth, if not the fictional arch is the metatarsal arch. Each will be dealt with in this obsession we have to talk about the foot and its arch.

The Longitudinal Arch

It was not until Harris and Beath set up a large study looking at 3619 Canadian soldiers' feet in 1947 that more information was forthcoming. They developed an ink mat to study pressure and arches, forming an arch index measurement.

> "It is a useless waste of time, effort and money to enlist men whose feet will not permit them to undertake the duties of a soldier even though they may have succeeded in finding themselves a niche in civil life in which they can compete on equal terms with their fellows."

This authoritative quotation comes from the classic and oft-quoted Army Foot Survey[21]

> "It is evident that we cannot be content merely to recognise the deformity of flat foot. Our concern is with function. If this is good it matters little whether the longitudinal arch is depressed."

With the exception of the cavalry, where most soldiers were not expected to rely on transport, an army depended on the foot soldier,. The reliance on feet and the ability of recruits to carry heavy loads on their backs required the army doctor to focus on the shape of the foot. Stories like the hunter-trapper made the exclusion of flat feet somewhat fallacious.[22]

> "...the hunter who tramped 200 miles out of the bush in order that he might reach Edmonton [Canada] to enlist, and then tramped back again the 200 miles to his trapping ground after he had been rejected because of his flat feet"

Fellner[23] used e-talk to discuss the flat foot and Harris and Beath's work. He stated that,

> "The flexible, or hypermobile, flatfoot accounted for most of the flatfeet that they identified in their study population. This type was determined to be the normal contour of a strong and stable foot, and not the cause of pain and disability. No one before nor since then has provided scientific evidence to refute their claim, yet the controversy continues."

---

[21] Harris, Beath 1947 An Investigation of Foot Ailments in Canadian Soldiers, published in 1947
[22] Seiden, H 1992 Flat feet don't automatically mean bad feet. The Gazette (Montreal) 17 Oct 1992: J6.
[23] Fellner D, 2012 E-talk Flat feet, kids, the military and orthopedists – what the literature tells us

The foot is designed to cope with terrain variation and conceived as three arches. The ankle joint, together with the talus influences both the arch shape and function of the midfoot. The x-ray illustration shows a child's foot before full development. Gaps appearing between the white (bone) are cartilage (black) and will be replaced by adult bone when mature. Cartilage has no calcium and phosphate salts which absorb x-rays so without any reflection the area of cartilage appears black. Compare this to the mature foot - x-ray on p.65.

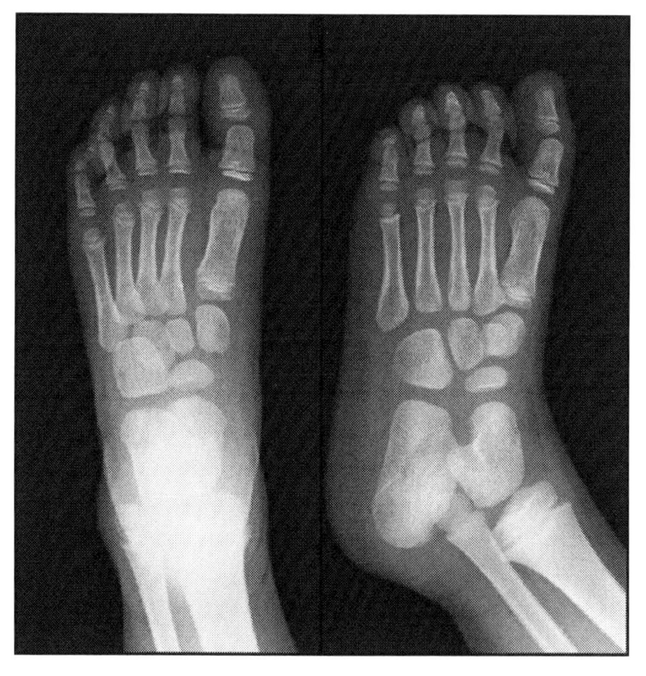

Altman (1968)[24] reviewed 138 subjects standing whilst x-rays were taken of volunteers aged 1-18 years. He drew lines on the films to show the different angles to the ground.

---

[24] Altman, M 1968 sagittal Plane angles of the Talus and Calcaneus in the Developing Foot. JAMA 58; 11:463-470

The pitch angle making up the long arch

The two bones that form the hindfoot, the talus and heel bone (calcaneus) are measured against the front of the foot. The angle called the pitch alters as the child develops. Without adding more complexity from this pivotal study, the shape of the arch changes with normal developmental foot growth. To study anatomy is glorious!

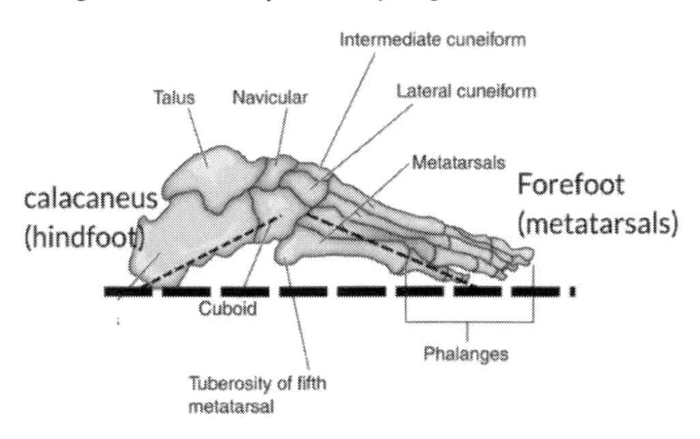

The diagram used above is for explanation and illustration and does not show the accurate line drawing that would be used if this had been a diagnostic study. Altman's study was large and unfettered by strict ethical approval. Today any research undertaken must be written up in such a way as to ensure that the benefit is clear and that no harm arises to the volunteer or co-workers. Altman's study was carried out in the USA and UK studies would more likely than not have used different permissible criteria.

The Transverse arch

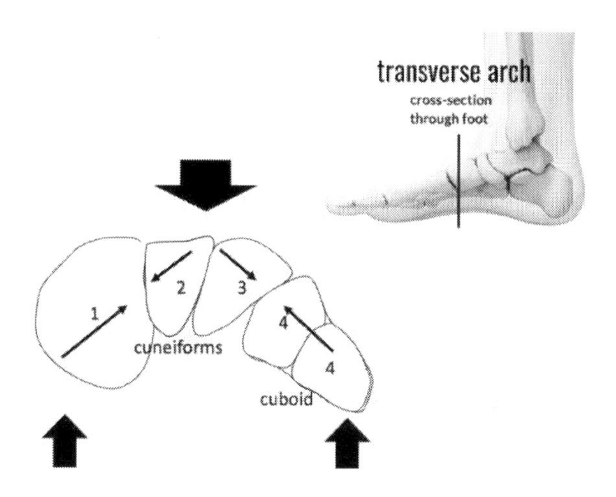

The transverse arch comes from a cross-sectional view of the middle part of the foot demarcated by wedge shaped bones. Made up of 3 cuneiforms and 1 cuboid, these bones fit the concept of the humpback bridge in cross section and arise in the midfoot. Their small interlocking joints fit like the bricks in the centre of the bridge. The foot would still maintain a theoretical arch without soft tissue to brace the bones. This fact forms a weak theory. However, if the large inside ankle tendon is cut, as occurred in a 8 year-old patient reported by Citron[25], the whole foot would collapse on the inner side. In dynamic terms, the bones act like square bricks. Body weight pushes down and the upward ground forces push the bricks together. As the body weight pushes downwards a band tightens making the foot arch stronger. This band is called the plantar fascia [fash-ee-ah].

---

[25] Citron's paper (1985) was a French case history, one I have always quoted to students in the eighties, but sadly could not locate.

As with most of these descriptions the pure mechanics have been simplified. High arch feet are less adaptable and in many ways are the opposite of the chimpanzee foot (p.64). The TT joint marked in the high arch shape is unyielding which is poor for walking on uneven surfaces.

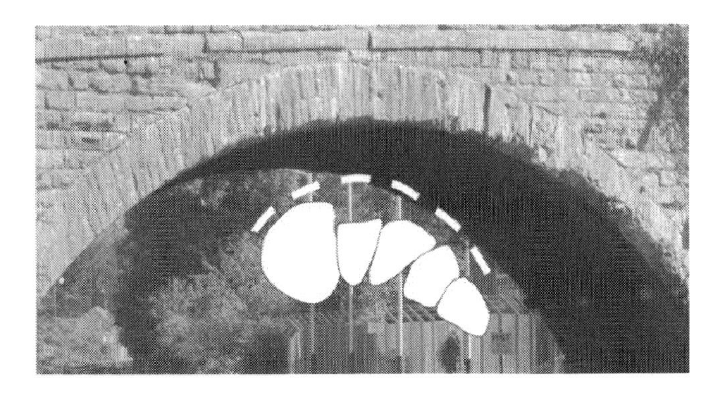

The vertical stones making up this railway arch have a similar mechanical-structural design with the mid-foot bones shown in cross section. The stability comes from the wedge shaped structure that not only interlock but use natural reaction forces (as shown in the previous diagram) to good effect. It should not be lost on the reader to see five surfaces illustrated under the bridge when anatomically there are only four bones. The two outer bones are in fact one bone (cuboid). There are two surfaces on the cuboid bone which allow the base of the 4th and 5th metatarsals contact. Check out the anatomy (p.15) if the bones do not make sense immediately. No-one said anatomy was easy!

As an aside, high arch feet do exist and that longitudinal arch and transverse arch can be sufficiently high enough to allow your fingers to pass through. Check the print left after walking in the sand or the bathroom floor to see what arch shape you have? Higher arched feet tend to be more rigid than low arched feet.

Is there such a thing as a dropped arch?

The mythical metatarsal arch

It is essential to say something about the *dropped arch*. This brings me to the third of those so called arches, the metatarsal arch. Unfortunately some authors mix the terms up so the transverse arch may be considered to be the anterior arch. Anterior is an anatomical positional term. If the ball of the foot is anterior then the heel would be posterior.

Forefoot (metatarsal heads)

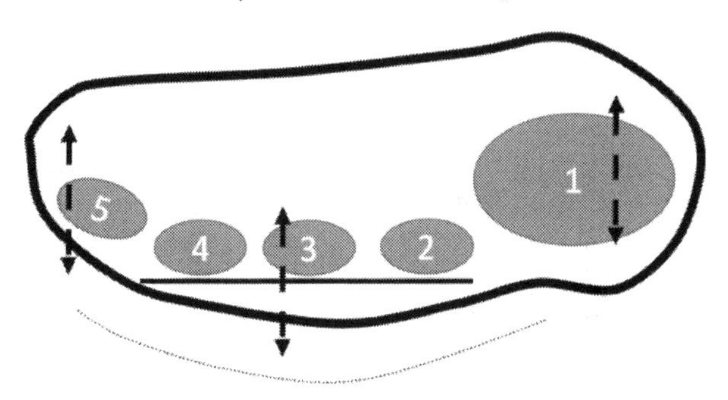

Ball of foot appears curved 'dropped'

The metatarsal arch above has been simplified to represent the ball of the foot. The three middle metatarsals work independently to the outer first and fifth metatarsals - solid horizontal line '2-4' works as one. There is no such thing as a dropped metatarsal arch but the longitudinal and transverse arches can alter in time with injury and disease.

Out of five metatarsals, the outer 2 (1 & 5) can rise up and down independently. Soft tissue, made up of fat and skin provides the impression that a metatarsal head has dropped in the centre, but this is an unreliable observation because the dropped appearance may be associated with a sac of fluid rather than bone; bursa or ganglion. The fine dotted lines represent this apparent impression seen by the eye.

Checking evidence for the metatarsal arch

The cross-sectional shape has always been difficult to capture by ordinary x-rays, although computerised scanning offers greater accuracy as it can make sectional cuts providing excellent images. Like everything in medicine this comes with a cost and the benefit to the patient must be justified. Magnetic imaging (MRI) is better than Computerised Tomography (CT) as the latter uses heaps more radiation than ordinary x-rays.

Suzuki did manage to take images from 100 feet, across this so called arch and 59 people with (bunions) hallux valgus, were compared to a control group[26]. The controlled group did not have hallux valgus. The heads of the central metatarsals showed little difference when compared. We draw the conclusion that the shape of this arch is illusionary and for the most part must be considered a myth. Suzuki calls the metatarsal arch the transverse arch. No wonder we are all confused about the arch.

[26] Suzuki, J, Tanaka, Y, Takaoka, T, Kadano, K, Takaura, Y 2004 Axial radiographic evaluation in hallux valgus: evaluation of the transverse arch in the forefoot. J.Orthop Sci. 9:446-451

What is fascia?

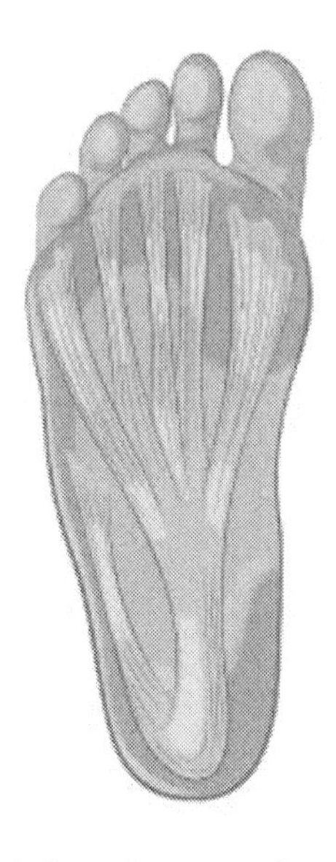

Have you ever cut the joint of meat so loved by British non-vegetarians? If you have then you will not only have seen fat running through red meat like veins, but the outer part of the joint has a shiny white covering. It is thin and tough for such a structure – this is the fascia. The main job of fascia is to act as support to other parts of the anatomy, especially groups of muscles. Fascia has a specific function in the foot and also known as the 'Windlass'. This means that as the band tightens, the forward fibres influence the toes. The band being thickest in the centre is tougher than muscle tissue. You are going to read more about fascia when we reach the topic - heel spur. During everyday active life we can cope with a flexible flat foot. However, if the tissues are exposed to strain, symptoms give rise to arch as well as ankle tendon strain.

Orthoses, a contoured arch filler (see in the next section), play a significant part in helping patients with these forms of tissue strain. Myths abound around causes of heel pain and inflamed fascia or fasciitis. It is true that fasciitis commonly arises in sports players. In 2019 an unstructured survey was carried out on 100 attendees at the Birmingham NEC sports conference and exhibition. The results suggested that plantar fasciitis was the number one topic that concerned runners[27].

Fascia arises in all the limbs and trunk, not just the foot, but it has little if no blood supply. Two fascial bands can become strained leading to significant discomfort, the foot arch fascia already mentioned, and the hip band or ilio-tibial band (ITB) on the *outside* of the upper leg[28]. Both can present with burning pain on movement. Unlike the fascial sheets that act as muscle group dividers, both the fascia in the foot and along the leg have more functional roles and can cause pain.

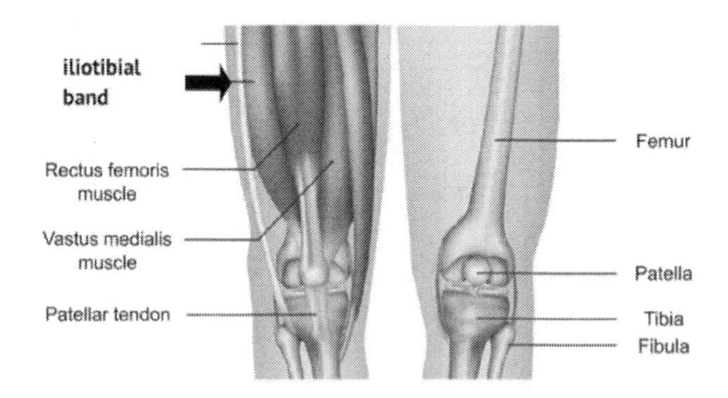

[27] The unpublished survey was carried out by a commercial firm with the help of this author as a pilot. Heel pain topped the responses..
[28] The diagram of the ITB is a schematic representation only

Arch supports called orthoses

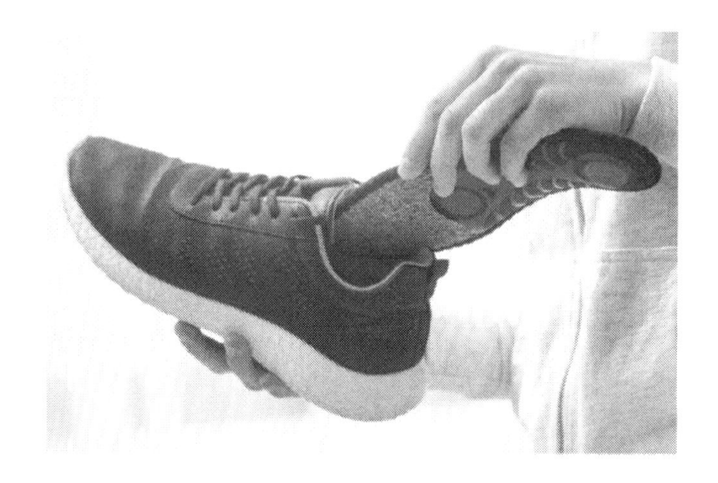

The low arch foot exists through normal development usually with a low pitched arch. This foot type has more flexibility. Some feet look flatter than others. Flat feet are common to black Caribbean races because the heel bone (calcaneus) has a lower pitch than in a Caucasian white person. Such a finding should not cause alarm. The Africoid association with the flat foot does not deter the individual from athletics as we know from success in the Olympics. However, if one believes a flat foot is a bad acquisition, then read on.

Shape changer - McPoil (2009) showed that the arch drops on weight-bearing by 14 degrees, and Nilsson (2012) by 13mm[29]. The length changes, as does the width with complete contact and provides shock absorption.

---

[29] Shekyhi-Dolagh 2015 (International prosthetics and orthotics international Vol 39(3): 190-96

Shock absorption comes from joints between the steering wheel bone (talus) and a boat shaped bone lying in front (navicular). The fascial band assists by bracing between the heel and toes as part of the Windlass Mechanism acting as a form of mechanical pulley. The foot leans in when we first contact the ground, then it comes back up bobbing like an angler's float on water as we move forward to toe-off. Without a trained eye, this subtle motion is only obvious when viewed when recorded and played back A flat foot will not necessarily tolerate a high arch support. This is a real problem and so finding an orthotic, often called an inlay, insole or appliance, makes life challenging.

Do flat feet need correcting?

Surgical management of the foot accounts for less than 5% of foot surgery performed in the UK[30]. Without pain, rapid shoe wear deterioration and increasing deformity in the foot, there is little justification for foot surgery. As far as performance is concerned, orthoses do offer better postural alignment. While the purchase of a pair of orthoses is harmless, prescription orthoses should be overseen by a trained professional. It has not been unknown for runners to cause extreme arch blistering by not building up time and distance slowly.

Shoe fit is the biggest problem when prescribing orthoses. Making a purchase, only to find that the device does not allow the foot to fit in the shoe, becomes an expensive problem. There are a number of different factors that determine the type of orthosis that a patient can tolerate. Females are frequently troubled by the limitations of shoe designs. The subject of the female shoe has its own section under footwear.

---

[30] PASCOM-10 database Royal College of Podiatry, London. This excludes data from orthopaedic contribution.

People with low arches may find orthoses uncomfortable and a disappointment without guidance. The golf-ball sensation is all too common if the shoe is filled up with thick material.

Research into orthoses

While there are many papers written about orthoses, Sheykhi-Dolagh's (2015)[31] paper highlights some of the reasons why some orthoses are not tolerated. Here are a few more facts from the study which forms the topic of evidenced based science/medicine.

Twenty people with flat feet aged 20-26 volunteered to randomly use three different types of orthosis. A rigid design, a semi-rigid prefabricated formed plastic and a softer orthosis (polyurethane) were selected as three choices.

Comfort was measured on a 1-10 scale, where ten was most comfortable. The rigid device scored three, the softer orthosis scored 6 and the semi-rigid orthosis scored 8. The semi-rigid orthotic was tolerated best.

Are rigid supports better?

Some foot control is better than no control, and soft materials do not make the best orthosis just because they are soft. Hard, rigid orthoses may control the foot better theoretically, but the arch cannot tolerate the pressure of some foot shapes. If your shop bought arch product doesn't work, then give a thought to your arch shape, joint deformity, flexibility and footwear design.

---

[31] Shekyhi-Dolagh et al The influence of foot orthoses on foot mobility magnitude and arch height index in adults with flexible flat feet. Pros & Orth. Int. 2015;39(30):190-196

Should feet be measured for pressure patterns?

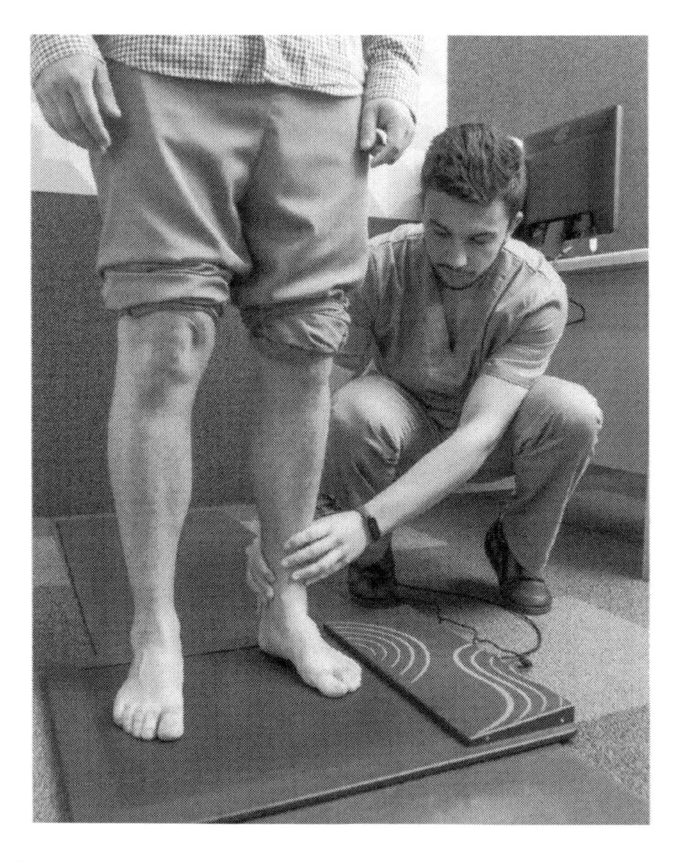

Much has been written about the arch and correcting the height, which cannot be done, but it attracts big business. The moral behind this tale might be, don't buy an arch support if your feet have no problems.

A growing market place, which ranges from random exhibitions to shoe shops, has sprung up in the 21st century with a strong sales pitch. The Health and Care Professions Council regulated the title of podiatry in the UK and other than nail care and pedicure, is limited to professionals. Foot Health Practitioners are often consulted and have their own voluntary body.

If I were to place your foot on a pressure platform and showed you an impressive graphic display, and then said if you purchase an orthotic it could help your posture and foot, you might be persuaded to purchase such an item.

Most adults have some aching in the musculoskeletal system at some point in their lives; back pain being common. We are a moldable agency which desires perfection and so many are easily persuaded by sales technique. There is no evidence that supports the mandatory use of any system to measure the foot to conclude a need for an orthosis based on nil symptoms. The interpretation of any pressure print is difficult to equate to specific conditions unless it is undertaken on reliable equipment and under scientific controls.

As equipment costs have dropped, the portable computerised pads are accessible to many non-medically trained people.

The science of pressure studies dates back to at least 1947 [32], although in the late seventies the first measurable studies emerged. Hutton and Drabble in 1972 made a significant breakthrough in the measurement of feet.[33]

---

[32] Schwartz, RP, Heath, AL. The definition of human locomotion on the basis of measurement (with description of oscillographic method) JBJS 1947;29(1) Jan.

[33] Hutton, WC, Drabble GE an apparatus to give the distribution of vertical load under the foot. Rheum. Phys.Med. 1972;11:313-317

Equipment accuracy has always been a problem. The technological side is excellent with measuring devices now at their best. However each walk through has to be taken several times to average out the best data.

The person undertaking the assessment must control variations from clothing to speed of contact. The variability in foot shapes and patterns is wide and it is easy to make assumptions.

The Electrodynogram (Langer US) was reported on Tomorrow's World, (a highly regarded science programme on BBC which ran for 38 years). The Electrodynogram was highly complex and was soon superceded with newer developmental concepts. The interface between the skin and shoe, the shoe and ground and the foot and ground make accurate measurement very difficult. The downward or vertical forces were soon recognised as not representative of real contact. The real make up of forces acting on the foot arise from three directions not a single direction. The fancy name was called orthogonal planes – sagittal, transverse and frontal planes.

Practices employing the latest equipment can show the centre of pressure and the direction of pressure but no reliable study can determine that an orthosis is mandatory. Pressure platforms exist to support skilled practitioners in their diagnosis and do not provide a diagnosis on their own merit.

The true value of measuring gait

The above criticism does not apply to scientific gait laboratories where they employ both pressure measuring platforms (force plates) and optical cameras which synchronise movement.

The use of such systems becomes very important in the prosthetic industry where injuries alter the balance of posture. Prosthetic limbs in the 21st century have been much influenced by brutal wars where IUDs have ripped off limbs but leave the broken human behind.

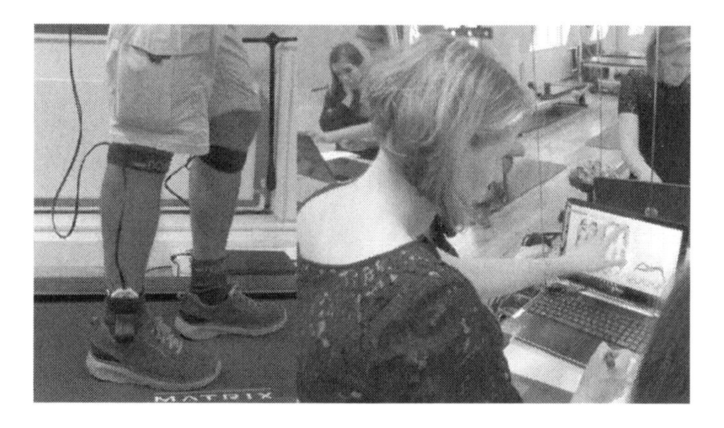

The professional seen above is using a commercial product to evaluate the author's pattern of walking. The pressure is measured using a sensitive insole connected to leads running to a back pack and then recorded in colour as part of computer software.[34]

Development continues to improve our understanding of pressures in the area of ulcer formation and changes made by deformity. The myth comes from the suggestion that non-professionals can make decisions. The fable emerges from a false moral assumption that patients need orthoses based on commercial products used as a selling tool. The fact lies with the need for evidence that such equipment is used both professionally and ethically. Lack of regulation exposes the consumer to a modern form of charlatanism now called capitalism!

---

[34] Courtesy of T D Prior and S Speirs (shown). The author's legs and feet are on the left hand side of the picture.

Tailors and the 'bunionnette'

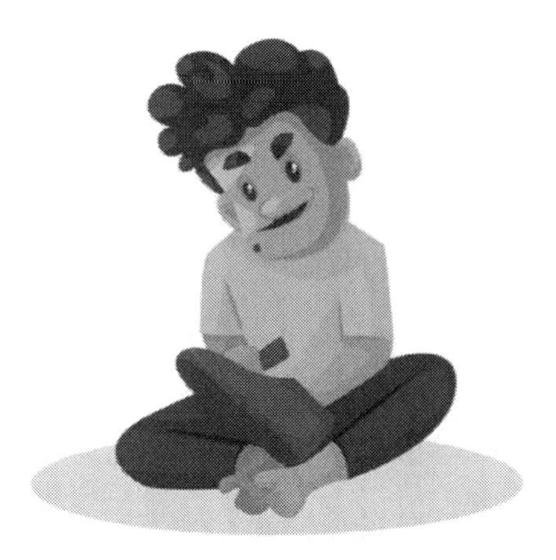

As we will learn later, many foot conditions are named after occupational titles. In the case of the tailor, he has been used to name the bump on the outside of the foot.

The myth surrounding the picture of the cross-legged artisan is just that because those suffering from wide feet often have both a bunion (see next) or a bump on the side of the great toe as well. The fact that sitting cross-legged will exacerbate the condition is indeed true. As with any activity, tipping the foot outwards will press on the soft tissues causing inflammation. 'Bunionnette' as a name for a small bunion seems apt, but as we will see with the first toe, this can be associated with deformity (dislocation) or a bony prominence.

Footwear selection should take account of the foot width. The tailor's bunion is more troublesome because it impacts on many activities, has an independent movement around the fifth metatarsal which lends instability to the side of the foot, and is often troubled with a ganglion. Read on to find more about bunions and ganglionic swellings.

Do only older people get a bunion?

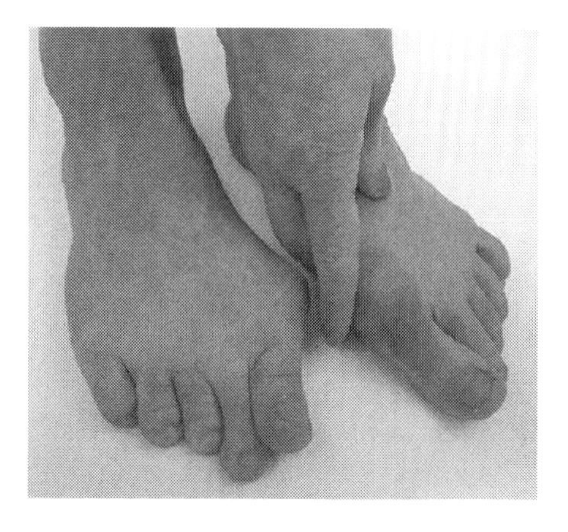

The deformity tends to start from thirties onwards but there are cases of the deformity being active in younger people. Older people just present with the end stage effects and this is where the greater problem with symptoms can arise. The subject is a massive one, such that I have committed it to a stand-alone book[35], but the reader will find plenty to read about in this chapter. The bunion, also known as hallux valgus, shares similarities with the tailor's bunionnette, which in the case of the latter, is smaller but no less of a problem.

Bunion may have derived from French, so the story goes. The word '*oignon*' means bunion, while in East Anglia (England) '*bunny*' means lump. The bunion is the bump and associated with extra-bone (exostosis) on the one hand. On the other, it is associated with a sac of fluid – ganglion.

---

[35] Tollafield, DR. Bunion Hallux Valgus. Behind the Scenes. Busypencilcase Communications 2019. Available from Amazon

How do we know if it is a bunion?

There are two tests

Test 1 - place your finger over the lump and see if your finger causes an indent. In other words, is it soft and spongy? If yes, it is a ganglion. If not, it is an exostosis because a hard sensation suggests it is a bony bump under the skin (p.86). You have to decide if it is a bunion or hallux valgus (bent big toe outwards).

Test 2 - place your hand over the bump so it is completely covered but leave the big toe end visible. If the big toe is straight and not pushing against the second toe, you have a bunion and not a hallux valgus. If the toe is bent and pushing the toe over, then you have a hallux valgus.

Is there a difference between a bunion and hallux valgus?

Bunions affect around 25% of the population, but this is a bit of an estimate. It is easier to call all toe problems with a large lump on the side of the big toe - a bunion. In truth, you can experience bumps on top of the big toe joint. So sideways bunions are called *medial* and top side bunions, *dorsal*. Sideways bunions have more joint movement than topside bunions. The latter has less movement related to the production of a bar of bone. Go to page 90 to see the range of hallux valgus deformities.

The extra bone (exostosis) is produced by the stretched ligament pulling inside the joint causing new bone growth.

The soft swelling is a thin sac of fluid, sometimes due to a bursa and sometimes a ganglion arising from damaged tissues associated with the joint lining change creating fluid inside an organised membrane or sac. The sac protects the joint on the one hand from further pressure until it becomes too large to fit into shoes.

Technically the soft sac associated with a ganglion and bursa are different if we look under the microscope. Ganglia have thin membranes and bursae have thick fibrous capsular outer membranes. Under the microscope bursae are usually anatomically normal while ganglia are not (p.157). Hard bunion prominences cause more of a concern if the skin is broken, leaving an open wound. If you are not good at healing, an ulcer may form due to constant pressure.

Older people suffer from bunions more than younger people, but this is not the case with hallux valgus, and can be seen from teenage years. There have been records of babies born with a hallux valgus, which is rare. As a clinician I have seen a case in a 9 year old where this particular deformity would have suited someone much older.

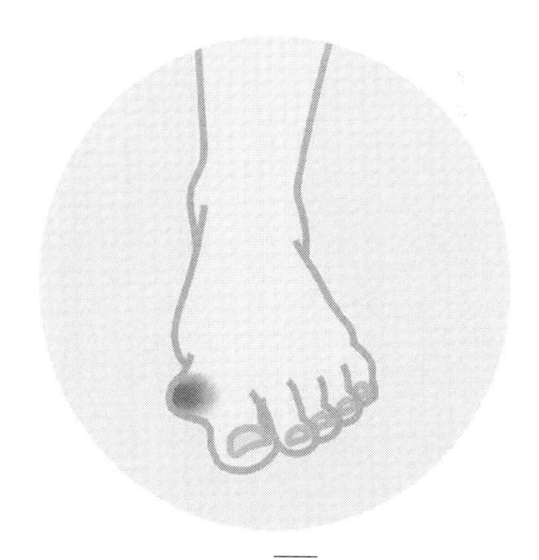

Is it true you can make a ganglion disappear?

We have seen the ganglion related to a bunion, but the ganglion can arise over the top of the foot and side of the ankle. The thin gossamer lining has a thick clear fluid-like gel. The lining is often hard to preserve during surgery. Internal degeneration arises and the formation of scar tissue creates an organised cyst. It is possible to draw fluid off a ganglion, but such effectiveness is more often short-lived.

One of the most interesting myths through time is the idea that hitting a ganglion with a heavy book reduces the swelling. The Bible, being the heaviest book in most older households, once upon a time, was a popular source. The Bible might have worked well if additional trauma did not lead to fractures! Ganglia and bursae often appear together in conversation. They are different although present similarly as visual swellings under the skin.

A heavy book will cause the outer membrane to burst. Reformation of any membrane can return if the derivative tissue remains. To complicate matters ganglia form from both joint linings and tendon sheaths. Ganglia can establish their structure within tendons[36]. A ganglion, when hit, can disperse, but the lining does not disappear and can regenerate within weeks.

Using a Bible was a representation of an accessible book and has nothing to do with religion. As the anecdotes came from a time when the UK was predominantly Christian, other representative religious groups were not mentioned as in the Koran (Qu'ran – Moslem), Torah (Judaism), Tipitaka (Buddhism) or books (poems) used by Hindus.

---

[36] Kono, M, Miyamoto, W, Imade, S, Uchio, Y 2009 Intratendinous ganglion in the extensor digitorum brevis tendon. J Orth Science Japan. 14:666-668

In modern parlance there are plenty of sources of heavy books but any form of hitting tissue is not recommended and certainly avoid using computer tablets and i-pads in place of the Bible!

Ankles, tops of feet, side and top joints of feet and even the toes have these swellings, although in the toes this is usually known as a mucoid cyst. While harmless, all swellings should be checked and treated by a specialist rather than a GP in many cases. Of course this depends on access to a professional. Ganglia descend deeper toward the joints and simply sucking off the fluid alone is pointless long term.

More bunion myths

One of the most frequent complaints that can come into the podiatrist's office is the bunion. We have three myths to solve.

- Provide evidence that bunions are not caused by footwear.
- Suggestions that you can use toe splints to straighten bunions.
- Decide if bunions are hereditary.

The most revealing picture in a podiatry textbook was a proud male of African descent standing for a photo[37] unshod. The tribesman had never worn shoes in his life and yet he had a sizeable bunion. The deformity was considerable and the forefoot was wide. Poor footwear can aggravate a deformity to reveal problems across the whole forefoot. Shoes alone do not cause the bunion. The skin becomes irritated over the bump causing localised damage.

---

[37] Root, M,L, Orien, WP, Weed, JH Normal and Abnormal Function of the Foot. Clinical Biomechanics.. Clinical Biomechanics Corporation, Los Angeles. 1977,Vol. II Page 386

The authors used the figure below to indicate the visual appearance of several examples of progression of the deformity[38]. As the deformity progresses the smaller toes lose their function.

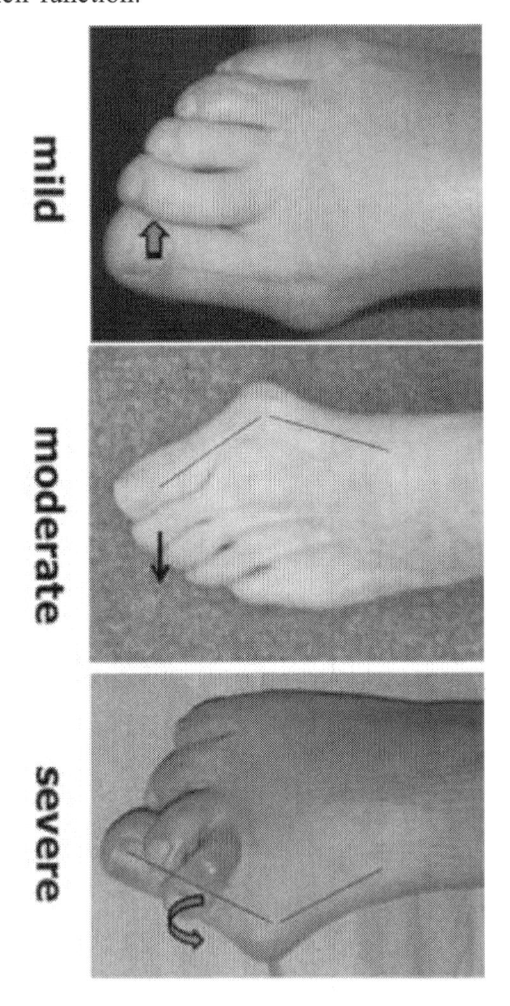

[38] Tollafield et al Clinical Skills in Treating the Foot. Churchill-Livingston/Elsevier 1997

Are shoes the cause of bunions?

Few studies examine multiple risk factors for hallux valgus although Nguyen (2010) considered a study involving a sample of community-dwelling older women and men in the USA[39]. One of the conclusions from the survey reflected the biological, structural and behavioural differences in men and women. Our cellular make up influences our behaviour from dress code to intersocial relationships. Nguyen considered that gender imposed different factors, borne out by twice the number of females to men that suffer. The role of body weight and height relationship (body mass index - BMI), high-heeled shoes and flat feet are all associated with foot pain in the presence of hallux valgus.

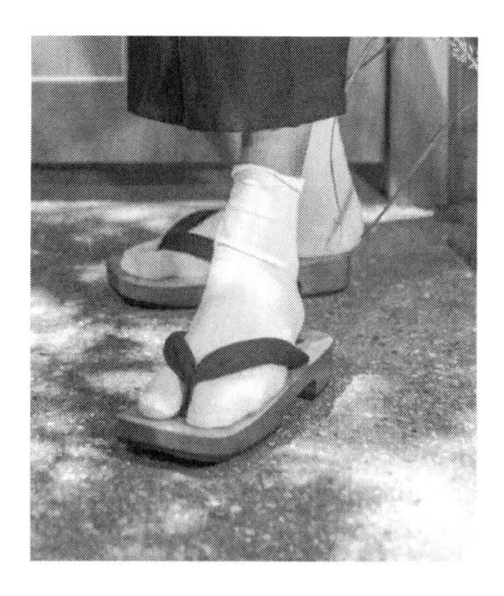

[39] Nguyen, US, Hillstrom, HJ, Li, W, Dufour, AB, Kiel, DP, Procter-Gray, E, Gagnon, MM, Hannan, MT. Factors associated with hallux valgus in a population-based study of older women and men: the MOBILIZE Boston Study. *Osteoarthritis*. 2010; 18 (1): 41–46.

Have Western Shoes Influenced Hallux Valgus?

A Japanese study (Kato 1981) considered that once the population had moved away from traditional shoe styles, involving Geta socks and Tabi sandals, in favour of western-style shoes, orthopaedic surgeons identified an increased incidence of operations.[40]

> "(The) incidence of HV deformity in Iranian university students, as a sample of Iranian youngsters, is much higher than those in some Western societies. This deformity showed to be highly inherent due to the increasing level of this deformity among first-degree relatives. Routine use of high heel or round tip shoes showed no influence on the rate of HV deformity." [41]

Davenport *et al*. (2014) added to the argument that HV does not come down to one factor alone.

> "Risk factors for hallux valgus… may include increasing age, female gender, genetic predisposition, constrictive shoe wear, first ray hypermobility, foot architecture, tight Achilles' tendon, and first metatarsal length." [42]

So, is it a myth that shoes cause bunions, given evidence from the findings of the Kato study? To understand a problem and use our scientific knowledge we have to consider more than one reading source.

---

[40] Kato, T, Watanabe, S. The etiology of hallux valgus in Japan. *Clinical Orthopaedics and Related Research*. 1981; 157: 78–81.

[41] Rahimi, A, Rezaee, M, Behrouzi, R, Naemi, S. Incidence of hallux valgus deformity among Iranian university students. *Ṭibb-i Tavānbakhshī*. 2012; 1 (2): 45–52.

[42] Davenport, KL, Simmel, L, Kadel, N. Hallux valgus in dancers. *Journal of Dance Medicine & Science*. 2014; 18 (2): 86–92.

Toe splints and separators for hallux valgus

Many believe if you push the toe over and hold it away from the second toe, the deformity can be corrected. This is a total myth. Toe separators are frequently shown in adverts for home products chiefly to straighten the big toe. Splints are also used after bunion surgery, although it is doubtful many foot surgeons (including this one) believe them necessary. Softer designs are for use in shoes, while the stiff types are for nighttime use only. Several studies, including Tehraninasr (2008), have been undertaken, but more recently, Karabicak 2015[43] and Plaass 2019[44] come to the same conclusion. Many advertisers stretch the value of splints showing models with perfectly straight toes. Splints work but only aid discomfort for short periods. Tehraninasr found that pain from bunions improved for a short period of weeks, but the deformity did not change.[45]

<u>Fact</u>

Toe splints have no adequate corrective power. Overcoming the deforming forces of dislocation of the first toe joint and contractures, let alone changing bone, is impossible. The next topic covers 'heredity'.

---

[43] Karabicak, GO, Bek, N, Tifticki, U. Short-term effects of kinesiotaping on pain and joint alignment in conservative treatment of hallux valgus. J. Manip.Phys. Ther. 2015;38(8): 564-571

[44] Plaass, C, Karch,A, Koch, A, Wiederhoeft, V, Ettinger, S, Claasen, L, Daniilidis, K, Yao, D, Stukenborg-Colsman, C Short term results of dynamic splinting for hallux valgus — A prospective randomized study. Foot & Ankle Surgery. 2019 https://doi.org/10.1016/j.fas.2019.01.002

[45] Tehraninasr, A, Saeedi, H, Forogh, B, Bahramizadeh, M, Keyhani, M. Effects of insole with toe-separator and night splint on patients with painful hallux valgus: a comparative study. *Prosthetics and Orthotics International*. 2008; 32 (1): 79–83.

If your parents had a bunion, will you get one?

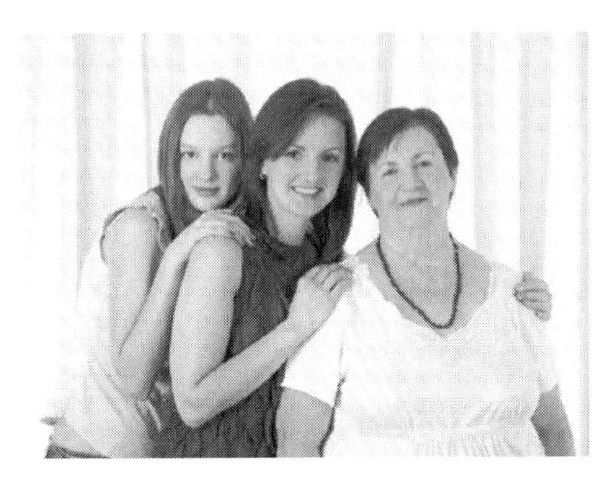

Without delving into Mendel's theories of genetic dominance we can apply some practical observations. Two matters jump out at us. Females suffer more from hallux valgus than males. The bunion can arise on the side or top of the big toe joint. Men certainly have bunions but cope better in male footwear. My grandfather's foot distorted the shoe comfortably! My mother had hallux valgus, as did her younger sister. Their mother died when I was ten so I do not know if she had a hallux valgus. My sister has the same problem, I don't.

Take the population of any country and females will dominate the bunion problem but also suffer more. If a parent has a deformity, then there is a reasonable chance you will have the condition. The only concern is how far will the problem progress? I have seen mothers and daughters with hallux valgus and this can affect one or both feet.

However, the gene can also miss a generation, so the grandmother can present with the problem and then the granddaughter.

Piqué-Vidal (2007) reviewed 350 subjects across three generations. The ratio of women to men with bunions was nearly 15:1 and provided a genetic line of argument as a 56% likelihood.[46] "The female sex predominated with regard to the gender of parents with *hallux valgus* … (the) severity of *hallux valgus* was not significantly influenced by gender, the affected branch of the family, or gender of the affected relatives. Family history of bunion deformity was present in 90% … affecting some family members across three generations, which is compatible with autosomal dominant inheritance with incomplete penetrance."

How bad can a bunion (hallux valgus) get?

The picture on p.96 shows that the first toe can continue drifting with age, but, although very rare, it is possible to be born with hallux valgus, a little known fact. The bunion is the enlarged area attributed to bone outgrowth (exostosis). Hallux valgus is a positional dislocation. Of course, the word bunion is misconceived and, in layman's terms, has various connotations. The reasons given for seeking help include,

> *"should I wait until it hurts?"*
> *"... don't like the look of it!"*
> *"want to stop it getting like my mother's"*
> *"can't get shoes on I want.*

The family doctor often sees a bunion differently, *not being ripe enough for surgery!* The bunion causes wide feet and alters the action of tendons, so hammer toes and dislocations misalign the forefoot. Grandparents who seek

---

[46] Piqué-Vidal, C, Solé, MT, Antich, J. Hallux valgus inheritance: pedigree research in 350 patients with bunion deformity. *Journal of Foot & Ankle Surgery*. 2007; 46 (3): 149–154.

no treatment may appear to have awful feet. My grandfather's shoes had that prominent bump, but the foot didn't hurt. His shoes were spacious.

Tight shoes will rub over fixed deformities, and pain adds to the discomfort. There is a litany of problems from corns to chilblains, ulcers to infections around the joint. The illustration shown below is by no means the worst foot but as the foot width increases dramatically, shoe fit becomes a trial. If toes dislocate then DO get an opinion as matters won't be solved alone. The hallux or great toe forces the smaller toes to dislocate (p.90). Overcrowding toes and deformities do tend to occur toward later life from 50 years onwards as a generalisation.

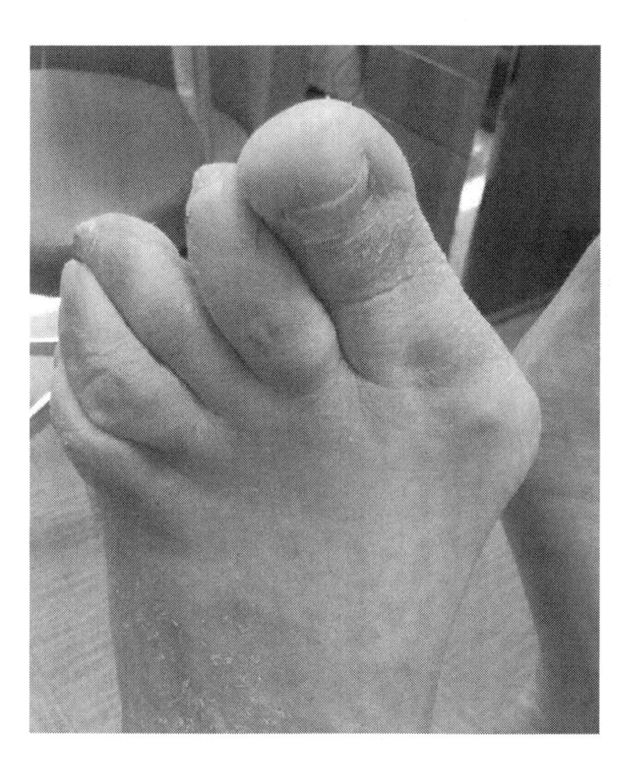

4 – Infection

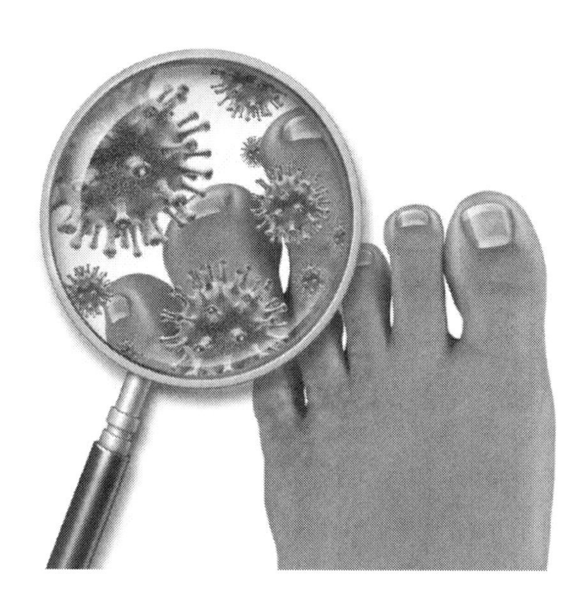

Infection is a word that can terrorise people, but is understood by the modern world more than ever.

It seems strange that we knew so little about the condition that brought bubonic plagues regularly to medieval populations and decimated armies. It took medicine into the late 18th century to make progress and another hundred years to find microorganisms responsible for infection. It was not until the end of the 19th century we understood viruses.

We have already met trench or immersion foot under 'skin', but there are some common and not so obvious infections worth highlighting in the foot. Under foot and mouth we learn a focal infection can appear in a different location to the original source. This is true in young patients where bone infection occurs through the blood stream. The moral of any tale associated with infection is to never ignore a child who complains of pain.

- What is infection and its signs
- Killing infection
- Foot warts
- Hygiene & sweat
- Athlete's foot
- Sugar and diabetes
- Peripheral neuropathy
- Chilblains& hot water!
- Trench Foot
- Elephant foot

Some of the other sources of infection have been left until the chapter on pain.

We all know what infection is – right?

An infection is a change in a wound that turns nasty and is attributed to micro-organisms. It may amaze readers to think that before the English surgeon, Joseph Lister, changed the face of medicine and surgery in Scotland, medical men of the day liked to apply dirt to wounds. Today the thought of dirt in open sores would be abhorrent. Bacteria were the main source of infection then and in hospitals they remain the number one problem. However, viruses interfere with our immune system as much as bacteria thrive without a healthy body to fight the process.

The product of infection from bacteria is pus. Pus is the result of the activity of the body fighting off anything that should not be present. White blood cells (remember the red cells carry oxygen) produce a lot of dead material after a battle with bacteria. There is just one problem that every clinician has to recognise. Pus or purulent discharge is not always infected. This means that the coloured thick or thin liquid may grow nothing – it is in effect sterile.

Is pus always a sign of infection?

While the body fights bacteria which in turn produces pus – a coloured discharge - in some cases this comes from the debris associated with white blood cells cleaning up unwanted bugs. Specialised cells are given the wonderful name phagocytes and are scavengers - the vultures of the African savannah, the maggots that clean up old food and detritus left behind as waste. The circumstances when this occurs in the foot depend on several factors. Pressure and blood supply. Let me explain.

If sufficient pressure is created across soft tissue, mainly skin and fat, then the living cells that make up our body tissue dies[47]. The resultant pressure from being squashed starves the cells of oxygen because the small blood vessels are damaged. When the threshold of normality changes, out come the scavengers and start cleaning up. As they do, they leave an untidy mess and if that mess becomes too large it does two things. This cellular debris is either pushed deeper into the foot, forming an abscess, or it will find a way to come to the surface, aided by chemicals (enzymes), to burst through the skin at the weakest point forming an unpleasant looking leakage.

One of the roles of a podiatrist is to remove the top layer and check the source and pathway of any infections or debris. A small exit hole may have a track called a sinus that needs exploring. Abscesses need draining because if left they will cause more damage and start to make the body ill. Abscesses that press on muscle make for bad news as death of muscle sets up other problems.

We can conclude then that the presence of pus is not always due to an infection but it is just as vital to have the foot checked out.

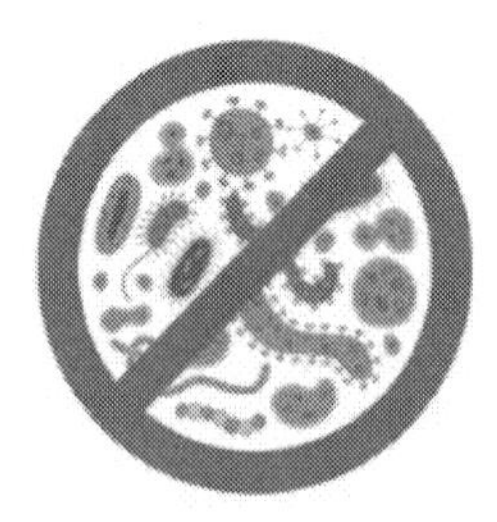

[47] Death of cellular tissue is called necrosis. Wet gangrene is infective as opposed to dry gangrene which arises due to loss of blood supply. Wet gangrene causes mortality.

Killing infection?

The three A's

Antiseptics, antibiotics and autoclave make up the three A's in fighting infection although clinicians would add asepsis[48] *as a fourth protocol.*

If antibiotics are not as useful for local wounds then why not use antiseptics? Antibiotics have disadvantages associated with allergies causing bug resistance and stomach upset. Why would a steriliser not be better than a solution of antiseptic liquid? All may not be as it seems. At my training college, we had to change from Dettol (chloroxylenol) to Hibitane (chlorhexidine). Dettol was growing the deadly Pseudomonas bacteria!

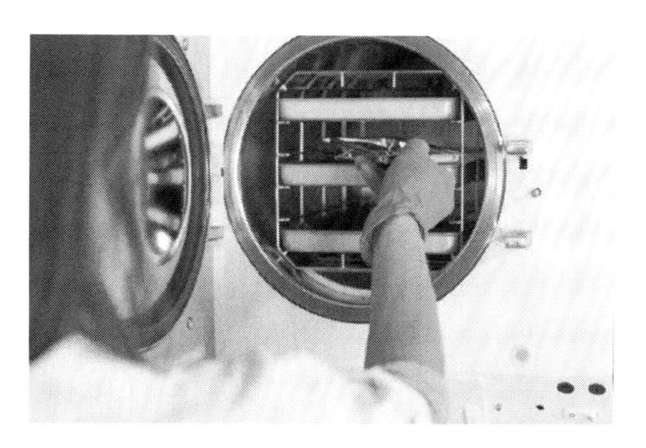

---

[48] Asepsis implies avoiding human contact with any foreign material. Gloves, masks and sterile dressings and equipment are prepared by various processes from autoclaves to irradiation. Asepsis is heightened by our awareness around PPE – personal protective equipment - to protect patient and carer.

Of course, an advert says that this former named antiseptic kills 99% of germs which sounds reassuring. But consider this, if the 1% of germs are not killed and carry significant harm, meaning if it gets into the body and thrives, well, the rest is bad news.

Before hepatitis B and AIDS/HIV were identified, viruses were still known to cause significant disease. Resistant to many treatments, viruses succumb to heat. Clinicians take no chances and throw the best methods called sterilisation at the bug, be it a virus, bacteria, fungus, protean or prion based infection.

A curious podiatry study

In this curious study conducted in 1979[49], I experimented with four methods of bug-killing media. The autoclave was the top of the tree as the only steriliser, while disinfectants included hibitane solution and formaldehyde. The last method was called a control. This is where no intervention took place and consisted wiping the same instrument without any other intervention. Sterilisation means killing 100% of germs, and disinfection means reducing the population of those bugs. The aim is to destroy all harmful organisms. You cannot autoclave a wound, so antisepsis and disinfection still must co-exist. Here is the conclusion from the study which was not published at the time the work was conducted as it had been intended as an internal review. *"Hibitane and formaldehyde perform similarly, while the autoclave performed less effectively, although the margins associated with percentage difference were narrow. All methods recorded some outliers put down to operator error.*

---

[49] Tollafield DR, De'ath,M, Prior, D [Peer Reviewed by Nixon, S, Pooke,M & Reed PJ in 1979] published 2018. https://consultingfootpain.co.uk/wp-content/uploads/2018/10/Comparison-of-disinfection-techniques.docx

Hibitane was produced with careful attention to the correct strength, but incorrect dilutions and irregular replacement could increase liquid contamination. Aesthetically the autoclave is more presentable and theoretically harder to interrupt cycles. While effective, the formaldehyde cabinet was considered less attractive because of potential problems with sensitivities to the operator and environment."

These findings were interesting because they looked at one instrument, a set of nail nippers and a scalpel. The use of disposable blades, like sterile gloves, today is an expected minimum standard. This prevents cross-infection. We have all heard of how someone passes an infection onto someone else, hence masks, gloves and even social distancing.

Cutting down on waste

In many cases, sterile metal instruments have been used as one-time use alone. Outside the clinic this may make sense with infected wounds, but the system is costly and where instruments are not recycled the environment will suffer. In several cases, sterilisation was not achieved with the autoclave. Sometimes autoclaves cannot penetrate small areas without pre-disinfection using an ultrasonic cleaner. The truth behind autoclaves being superior is sound but the system is only as good as its operator. Additionally the equipment must be serviced and kept in good order with scientific testing. It is a fact that sterilising with autoclaves is important. Antiseptics cause fewer problems than antibiotics which should only be used in justifiable cases. Ultrasonic cleaners allow instruments to dislodge smaller particles[50].

---

[50]https://www.aegisdentalnetwork.com/ida/2010/09/cleaning-instruments-a-critical-step-to-instrument-reprocessing

Verruca

The word verruca is Greek for wart so foot warts are entitled verruca pedis. Pedis is Latin for foot. Language plays a big part in medical terminology.

It is probably a truism that this virus did more to allow podiatry entry into the world of child foot health, although much has changed over half a century under NHS provision. There are still many questions asked about this nuisance foot problem.

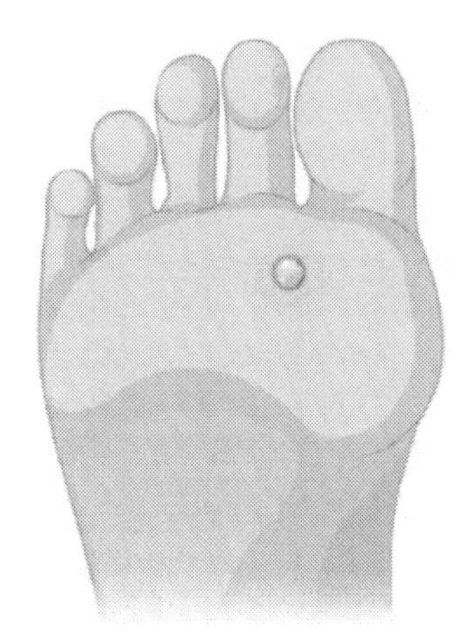

The location of the sole is more common for this infective lesion, often know as a plantar wart because the sole is called the plantar surface, much as the hand is called the palmar surface. Contrary to belief, warts are not ingrowing and do not have roots. We can all recall pictures of bent over witches depicted with warty projections from their faces and hands.

The schematic diagram is a typical appearance but in reality not all warts appear as well demarcated. Multiple locations, arise, grouped or diffusely spread warts (mosaic) all confound treatment. Those on toes and on top of the foot often project without the pressure of the ground.

The sole of the foot compresses the normal outgrowing skin pushing it into the deeper elements. If you have tried to remove a wart then there is a good chance it will have bled.

Warts are caused by a virus or Human Papilloma virus (HPV) and affect all parts of the body.

Sexually transmitted warts are different and do need early treatment. While foot warts rarely cause cancer, the virus can alter in some cases and genital warts are one such infection which can lead to cervical cancer.

wart (verruca pedis)

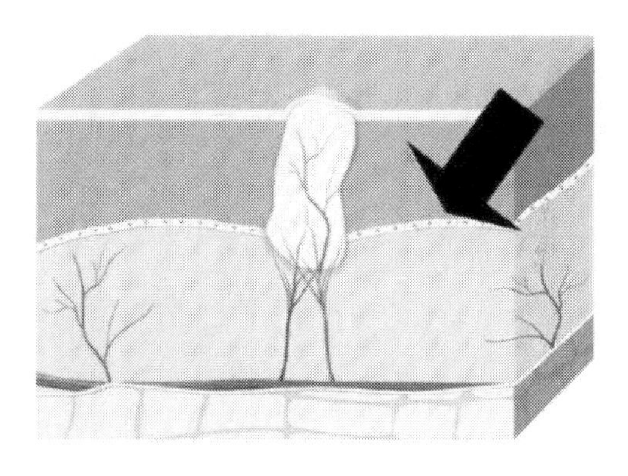

The infection alters the separating membrane between the top thick (inert) layer and the living layers (black arrow). The membrane is important for normal top layer growth. Over production of the skin cells causes callus and corns.

It is incorrect to say the skin is dead because of course it depends on a lower layer that is highly active. The layer beneath the epidermis is called the dermis and this is where the business end is, made up with nerves, blood vessels and cellular material able to fight infection. We might say that the skin is inert in the top layer. Like a medieval knight, his armour might protect him from most external sources but if punctured by an arrow the internal part will soon show signs of weakening.

Corns versus warts

Now here's a little known fact. Many painful corns are in fact mixed with this little virus which implies the two conditions co-exist. How do we know this? Full removal of all the skin and deeper tissue cells are examined under a microscope and show appearances typical of this virus. Unlike bacteria, viruses are smaller and can remain dormant for a long time with little change. Small vessels within the substance of the keratin give it a vascular appearance. It is not unusual to find a larger dark area of amassed cells signifying that the virus is all played out – or put simply, it is 'dead' and now inactive.

Can I get a verruca from a swimming pool?

The answer is yes, but such a statement requires qualifying. You will not get a foot wart directly from the water. There are far worse bugs that you can find in untreated water, but warts are not one.

You require two factors. A small crack in the skin; one you will not see and secondly you need a surface. Floors around pools and showers are often made of porous lining materials.

You cannot see these viruses under an ordinary microscope because these organisms are much smaller than bacteria.

Do plastic socks work?

Socks remove the first portal of entry and then protect the skin from further damage. Children have softer skin and are more prone to this infection. They also have weaker immune systems and like chicken pox (varicella) – another well-known virus – confer better immunity once infected.

Another little unknown fact is that the vaccination for smallpox (Variola) was shown to work on HPV infections, but because there was a fear of overuse of this innoculation, and smallpox was so feared, that, as with antibiotics, natural immunity is preferred. Smallpox left devastating scars and was eradicated by 1979. Vaccines do exist for HPV, especially to protect girls from cervical cancer, but as far as feet are concerned, the evidence has not been as conclusive.

Once infected can I get another verruca?

Once you have been infected you are better protected, but there are over 60 different strains of virus. It is possible to pick up a new strain, i.e a different HPV. I have had one verruca on my foot when young, but several on my hands when I was older. We are the better to resist warts as we age, but, they can be a nuisance. The second part of the answer is a little more disappointing.

Disease lowers our resistance and therefore immunity. Remember immunity is dependent on the white blood cells being able to mop up infection fast. We also need a good lymphatic system especially around the groin and arm pits and even bone, where some of the resistant fighting cells are manufactured.

Auto-immune diseases like rheumatoid arthritis diminish our ability to resist infection as is the case with infections like AIDS or leukaemia where white blood cells are either low or are ineffective in larger quantities. Therefore, further wart infections will depend on our health and state of mind. Let's look at that steak again from p.19

Can I bury a piece of steak in the garden to take my wart away?

No, this is a myth and of course expensive. It is also not directly possible to charm warts away but here is the conundrum. Belief and wellbeing can help our immune system. A stressful life does not help but holidays can. Many find warts simply go when the source of stress is removed. If you are hypnotized and you believe in the process then change may happen – but there is no guarantee I'm afraid.

Do over the counter products get rid of warts?

Like everything in life there is no *one* fix for all. Today, and not just because of our experience with Covid-19, we know race, age, genetics, disease and gender all make a difference to how we cope with illness.

At present we are still a little unsure what treatments are best for all these different racial and gender groups. A doctor specialising in problems of the skin is called a dermatologist, although the foot wart is part of health care delivery, warts are not treated under the British NHS as they were in the eighties. There is a belief that the infection is self-limiting and will go in time. Economy and costs will also drive decisions about what is offered on the NHS.

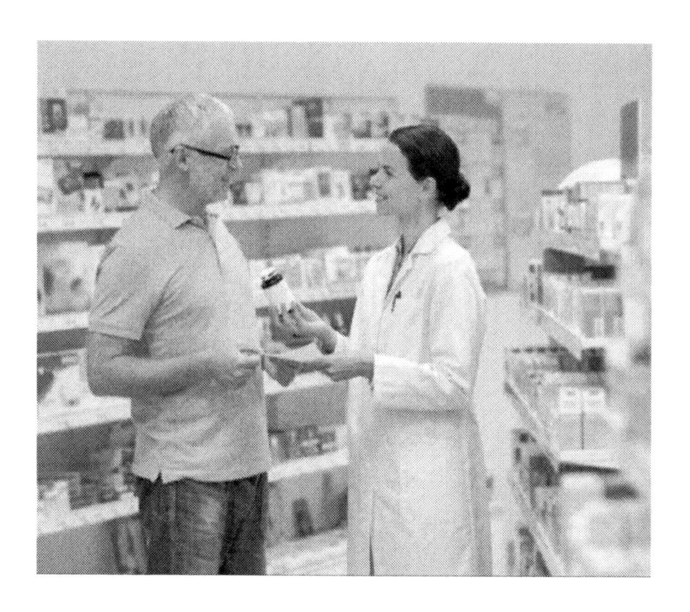

What works on a child up to age 16 may be different for an older person. Your pharmacist will guide you to the products but will not have expertise to guide you precisely in all the best foot treatments. Podiatrists still specialise in verruca management but many such infections can be extremely resistant to treatment. There are a wide range of remedies which include freezing and heat destruction.

Needling is a newer technique that has gained popularity amongst podiatrists. The wart is punctured so stimulating an immune response. Pastes and acids are useful but can create unwanted damage and scarring. This form of treatment is less favoured today, although plasters and pastes are still sold by pharmacists.

Hygiene issues and feet

Smelly dirty feet make up the biggest 'ugh factor' for the podiatrist and perception of what might be unsavoury. Like a funeral director or refuse collector it might not appear as an attractive profession but it is rewarding on so many fronts and makes a satisfying career. By and large smelly gungy feet are not that common and people care about odour in feet as much as they do around arm pits. There is usually a good reason why feet might suddenly appear unsavoury. Part of our role is to investigate the problem and then manage it.

Why are my nails dirty?

There are several good reasons why your nail is discoloured. Forget what happens to your finger nails when you work with dirty tools and products. Unless you are in the habit of going bare foot, or your shoe leaks when out walking, or is affected by the dye in your shoe – there is a cause. Toenails are no longer a valued part of our body as our finger nails are. Nails are weapons and tools of the trade on the four limbs.

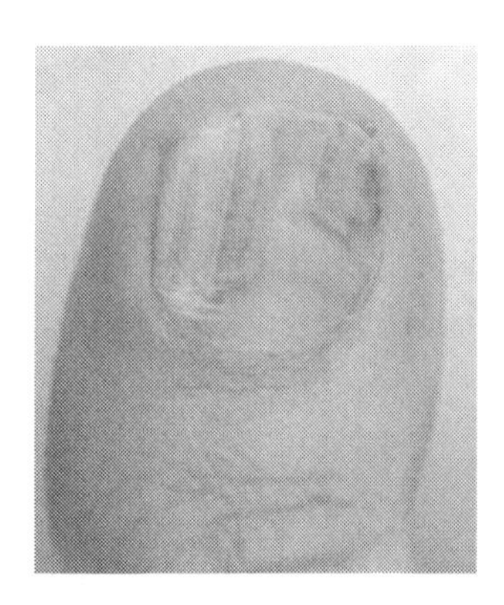

Unlike our pets we cannot scratch our ears with our feet in adulthood. The nail, like the skin is made from a protein called keratin. This is the same substance discussed earlier with corns and callus. Keratin is hard, resistant to water and keeps out those nasty bacteria and viruses. However, the nail ages and thickens with use. The quality changes in density and structure. A sporting or occupation such as dancing may rip a nail after prolonged pressure and initiates the process of repair and thickening. The nail lifts at the end and starts to separate. The gap left between the under surface of the nail and the skin leaves an entry to another bug – fungus. Think about stale bread forming penicillin-like-mould. Dark, warm and moist environments encourage the growth of fungal spores.

Fungi with names

We podiatrists love names and if we can grow a fungus bug from a nail sample we are thrilled and can tell our patients they have *trichophyton rubrum* or some other wonderful foreign name. Of course names are in Latin or Greek! Fungus the Bogeyman, inspired by the artist *Raymond Briggs* comes to mind. Perhaps we should talk about mycoses as a fungal infection is a mycotic infection as we see bacteria being a bacterial infection. The brown, yellow and even blue-green features are just bugs taking up their new home. They are opportunists as they see a chance for starting a family. As far as health is concerned fungi (mycoses) are not likely to endanger healthy humans. The nice look no longer looks so nice. Podiatrists used to reduce the keratin to treat these nails but today they should only do so with masks, respirators and with drills supported by dust extraction because those fungi spores can find their way into the lungs and that is no longer acceptable.

Cross-infection

Cross-infection is how we pass bugs from one person to another. We think of hands and of course breathing out germs. Closed in spaces with poor ventilation adds to the problem of inhalation. Using a nail file that has been contaminated means you push the same bugs onto the new *host*. The idea of cross-infection is well known and this is why we wash our hands as we do not know what we might pass on. Again, Covid-19 has shown that those with poorest health are at greatest risk from cross-infection. But here is an interesting fact - in cases of clean surgery, facemasks have not always been seen as valid at protecting against post-surgical infection[51]. It would be a brave person to take avoiding masks as a valid rule in this new age of rising infections.

Can I get dust in my lungs from filing my nail?

Research has been active since the 1970's in this regard[52]. The chance of this happening would be unlikely if you used a hand file. You have more chance of infecting adjacent toe nails than causing lung dust problems. However, try to file nails manually without drills. Ensure you have an aired open space. And, do not share nail files with anyone, even a partner.

---

[51] Tunevall, T.G. Postoperative wound infections and surgical face masks: A controlled study. *World J. Surg.* **15,** 383–387 (1991). https://doi-org.libaccess.hud.ac.uk/10.1007/BF01658736
[52] Workplace Exposure to Bioaerosols in Podiatry Clinics Coggins, MA, Hogan, VJ, Kelly, M, Fleming, GTA, Roberts, R, Tynan, T, Thorne, PS. The annals of occupational hygiene, Volume 56, Issue 6, 17 July 2012, Pages 746-753, https://doi.org/10.1093/annhyg/mer124

Do you have to be an athlete to get athlete's foot?

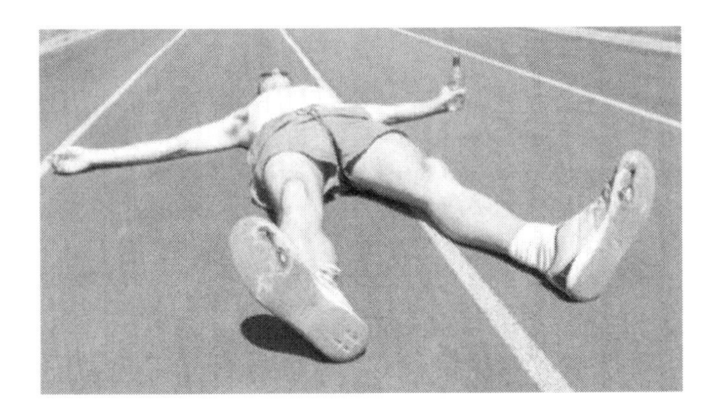

Skin can become infected with a fungal infection but the appearance is different from nails. Nails make a good substrate while skin behaves differently. Again the foot needs to create the right environment for fungi. Athletes commonly have skin problems assumed to be associated with mycotic infections. The heat and moisture produced by exercise activity can be impressive. Without the flow of air – some shoes now have holes to help – heat build-up requires the body to sweat. This moisture pools and soaks back into the skin causing softening. Athlete's foot, often known as Tinea Pedis, forms small blisters called vesicles which are itchy and can spread. In science we talk about the power of hydrogen or pH. The sweat can change its pH. The more hydrogen (H_2) the more acidic a solution, the less H_2 the more alkalinic. Sweat increases to help cool our skin temperature. The downside to this is that the foot becomes more alkalinic and prone to alter the types of bugs grown, attracting insects we don't want in our floral garden .

We find the alkalinity in sweat helps bacteria and therefore we don't want to attract anything that disturbs our balanced skin flora. Keeping the skin healthy without being too dry or moist is important. The oily nature of skin protects our skin as polish protects the bodywork of a car. In poor health the skin flora can change opening up the risk of other bugs affecting the skin. Healthy skin has a coating of friendly bacteria. *Staphylococcus epidermidis*, known as commensal flora, affords protection. Think of flora as a nice flower bed with mixed colours attracting bees. Now reverse that thought and say you don't want the bees to be attracted.

The problem with fungal infections, like bacteria, fungi like an alkaline medium and so bacteria and fungi can work together.

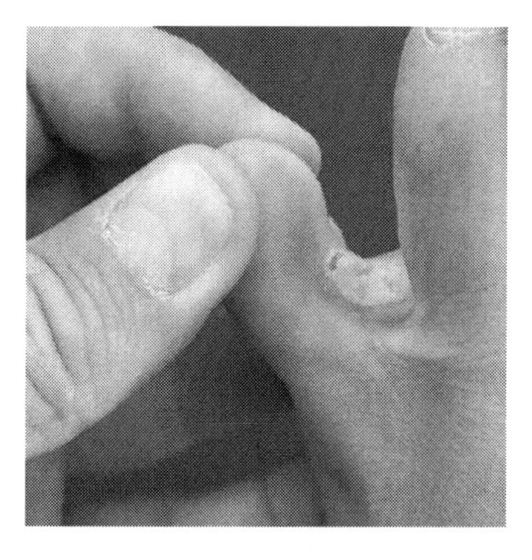

The skin is soggy, macerated and has an unpleasant odour but this is bacterial. However, treatment as athlete's foot should be considered together with improving the air circulation to allow this to dry faster. Sandals and open designed footwear work best in the right environments.

Mimicking Athlete's foot

"The patient looked down at his toe and saw flaky skin - white and raw. It itched madly, had an odour, and so it was assumed that dastardly condition toe fungus." See p.114

The condition of skin fungi has various names, including Dhobi's itch. The latter term relates more to the irritation found in the groin and areas where sweat builds up. Athlete's foot is more commonly attributed to this condition and has a fungal rather than bacterial origin. Athlete's foot (dermatomycosis) is associated with warm climates but can affect us in winter and summer because we fail to dry in an area susceptible to the problem. This annoying condition affects the small toe, or to be more precise, affects the inside cleft of the fifth toe. Full-blown fungal infections can have a ring-like feature (ringworm) and affect skin across the foot and other parts of the body. Blisters emerge as small vesicles predominate the sole and arch. Nails are also affected by fungus but may take much longer to arise and treatment is prolonged. The little toe or fifth toe has a cup shape indent toward the base as it connects with the foot. The cup acts to trap water if the area is not dried. The skin becomes soggy (macerated) and sets up an irritation within a short period If the skin surface (epidermis) sheds or flakes, the lower layer is exposed and cannot combat fungus or bacteria well. The change in odour is noticeable and confined to the scooped out shape. Often by the time the person notices, the problem has hatched. A small area of pooled sweat accumulates attracting the problem and yet it is easy to prevent by drying thoroughly after bathing.

Sweaty feet!

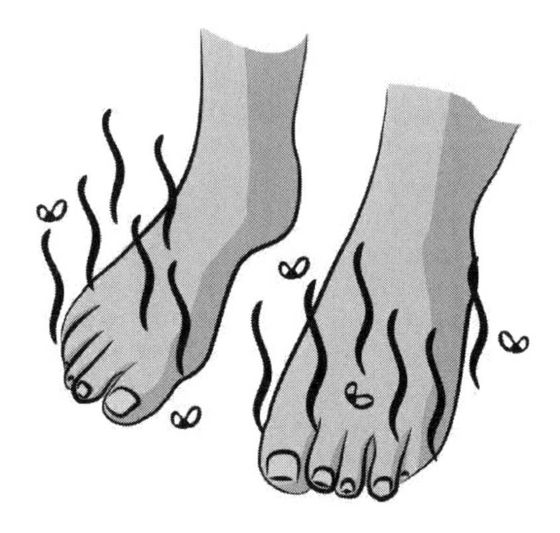

Are sweaty feet due to poor hygiene?

Few things put people off more than the thought of sweaty feet. According to one source, your feet have more sweat glands than any other part of your body – even more than your armpits. *"It's entirely normal for your feet to produce more than a pint* [568 mls] *of sweat in any given day, says Dr Juliet McGrattan in an article for netdoctor"*[53].

The term for smelly feet is *bromidrosis*. The term for excessive sweaty feet is *hyperidrosis*. But contrary to popular belief it's not the sweat that causes bromidrosis. Foot odour arises from the bi-product that bacteria produce,

---

[53] McGratton,J citing Andersen, F 2019 https://www.netdoctor.co.uk/conditions/infections/a5560/viruses-and-bacteria/

offering four prominent smells: sweaty, cheesy, vinegary and cabbage-y.[54]

> "Methanethiol is a key component in the flavor of cheddar cheese. Acetic acid is a result of sugar fermentation — and is better known as vinegar. Byproducts associated with rot, such as propionic acid and butyric acid, can leave feet smelling like rancid cabbage. The most common foot-related chemical, isovaleric acid, is responsible for the smell we call "sweaty." Our noses are up to two thousand times more sensitive to this chemical than the others, and many of us can recognise it even at the slightest concentration."

Bacteria live on the skin of your feet and digest the sweat, producing chemicals thought to be the cause of the smell. The sweat glands are also active in the hands as well as feet. The value of sweat, up to a point, allows some grip and traction as the skin is not smooth.

Sweat glands

There are 250,000 sweat glands in the feet. Some sources suggest our sweat glands, known as eccrine glands, may exceed McGrattan's statement and therefore the real quantity of sweat produced will depend on weather, activity or stress levels to start with. Nerves and hormones regulate this activity. Men sweat more than women.

Poor hygiene adds to the build-up of skin squames offering greater bacterial opportunity. However, increased sweating requires temperature, exercise, stress and can be affected by medical drugs and chemicals as in foods. Increased sweating may require medical intervention. One condition that is not so uncommon is pitted keratolysis. We

[54] Tetro,J Bacteria Give Feet 4 Distinct Odors March, 2020 https://www.discovermagazine.com/planet-earth/bacteria-give-feet-4-distinct-odors

have met the word 'lysis before which means to break down.

Corynebacterium or Kytococcus sedentarius are causes of this intense smell. The appearance is pronounced with pits made within the top layer of moist skin turned white. Contact with the skin and aroma make this highly offensive. Similarly, interdigital sweating (between toes) can lead to bacterial breakdown as in the case of toe irritation seen on page 114-15

Medical reasons for sweating

- Injury
- Infection (Tuberculosis)
- Emotional (psychological /mental/pain)
- Diabetes
- Increased thyroid activity
- Cancers (blood/lymph)
- Skin – pitted keratolysis, tinea pedis (athlete's foot)

Conclusion

Sweaty feet are usually unrelated to poor hygiene alone and may have more to do with a medical problem. Managing bacterial activity is essential, but the primary casualty is footwear. Good hygiene is still essential if this problem does exist.

Where foot conditions don't follow occupational names they might be named after medical men or animals. And so we meet the case of elephant foot.

Sugar and diabetes

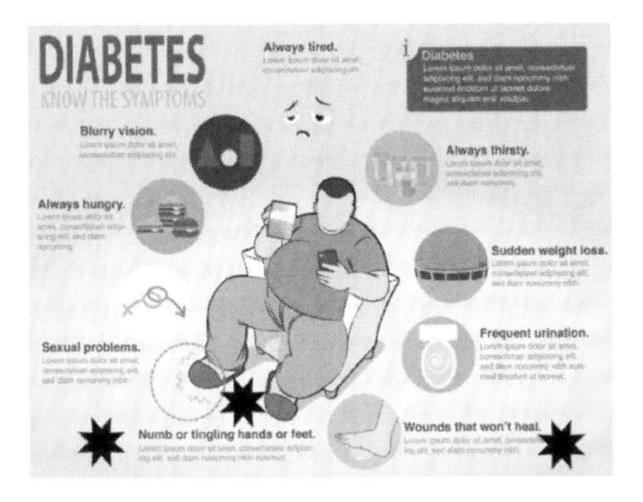

As a child I learned that my grandmother had 'sugar diabetes' and just assumed she had eaten too much sugar. I was only aged 8 at the time so completely unaware of the real process behind the disease. High blood sugar means that the hormone insulin is not working and when the blood sugar is elevated above normal, this is referred to as a hyperglycaemic state.

Sugar sweet feet

Podiatrists are concerned when the body's sugar digesting mechanism becomes unbalanced. This affects patients who suffer from one of two types of diabetes.

Type 1 is usually inherited and develops early on. In this case problems such as fungal infection may be more noticeable and give away the diagnosis. The cells that produce insulin are faulty.

Type 2 or late onset diabetes is different and can be corrected, but again the give-away signs may include athlete's foot. Two of the nine conditions in the publicity poster over the page concern feet and are marked with asterisks.

> "Around two million people in England are at risk of developing Type 2 diabetes, the highest on record, according to new NHS figures. The new figures come as the NHS ramps up efforts to treat, prevent and even put the illness in remission, as part of the NHS Long Term Plan. Latest stats show there are 1,969,610 people registered with a GP who have non-diabetic hyperglycaemia, a condition which puts people at high risk of Type 2, which is the highest on record. The scale of the problem is likely to be even greater as the growing obesity crisis is exposing millions more to the condition."[55]

Consider an open fire needing dry wood to make heat. If we store this poorly we won't be able to use the fuel until we correct the storage method. In some ways diabetes creates an inefficient method of using fuel, which in this case is sugar. We use insulin stored in the organ called the pancreas to access sugar efficiently from muscles and fat. The skin flora is altered in diabetics and a sugary mix makes a wonderful platform to attract all forms of bugs; mycotic and bacterial alike. So there is no myth about sugar, as high levels of unrefined sugar can cause the pancreas, the organ that produces insulin, to fail. Numb, tingling feet and poor wound healing form the key signatures of uncontrolled diabetes in feet.

Many other factors — including overall diet, lifestyle and genetics — add to the risk of developing diabetes. Studies have found that people who regularly drink sugar-sweetened beverages have an estimated 25% greater risk of

[55] https://www.england.nhs.uk/2020/02/record-high-two-million-people-at-risk-of-type-2-diabetes/

type 2 diabetes[56]. The link between sugar intake and diabetes can still arise even after controlling our calorie intake, body weight, alcohol consumption and exercise[57]. While these studies may not prove that sugar causes diabetes, the association is compelling.

Of course not all sugars are glucose. Fructose, another sugar that comes under the heading carbohydrate, promotes fatty liver. If you eat more sugar than your body can use for energy, the excess will be converted into fatty acids and stored as body fat. High intakes tend to increase fats which may increase your risk of heart disease and fatty liver. If all of this seems worrying, fructose is also associated with higher uric acid levels in blood. If the crystals of uric acid settle in your joints, gout can develop.

Weight gain is a common problem with increased sugar intake leading to morbid obesity and fat increase.

In some cases primary care doctors miss diabetes until it is established. This is not because they are bad doctors but screening systems can be patchy and it is worth pushing for a health screen at least once in five years after age 50.

Modern podiatry can act as a medical screen for many problems. These include detecting high blood pressure, advising on diet and obesity, as well as checking out skin conditions for malignancy. Another bonus for foot patients is the fact that new diagnostic equipment used to listen to pulses and circulation in feet and legs can also assist detect abnormal heart sounds. Podiatrists can play a significant part in helping monitor and solve early disease problems.

---

[56] Wang M, Yu M, Fang L, Hu RY. Association between sugar-sweetened beverages and type 2 diabetes: A meta-analysis. *J Diabetes Investig*. 2015;6(3):360-366. doi:10.1111/jdi.12309

[57] Basu S, Yoffe P, Hills N, Lustig RH. The relationship of sugar to population-level diabetes prevalence: an econometric analysis of repeated cross-sectional data. *PLoS One*. 2013;8(2):e57873. doi:10.1371/journal.pone.0057873

Does numbness matter?

Tied into risk, disease and infection is the body's own way of detecting harm. White blood cells are important for infection but the nerve pathway is equally as important. If we cannot feel when we harm ourselves the problem described previously can lead to ulcers, abscesses and wounds that fail to heal. While skin sensation is affected in a number of conditions it will also affect sensory information picked up by nerves in joints and tendons. Walking can alter as a result of neuropathy.

Specialised nerves

According to Neurogenetics at the University of Tennessee Health Science Center, the human body has 95 to 100 billion neurons or nerve cells[58]. Nerves serve many purposes, but it is the part of the nerve ending at the skin which alerts us to damaging temperature changes (heat & cold), excessive pressure that can cause harm, and sharpness when we tread on a pin or splinter. Should this detection system fail then we have a state called *neuropathy*. Toes and fingers are very sensitive and have more pressure sensors than the rest of the foot. Feet and hands are important radar organs. We also have dedicated pain sensors (nociceptors) in the body. Some parts of the body are more sensitive for a specific reason. The erogenous zones are packed with sensors to fire off the process of reproduction. We find the tongue provides another sensory function to serve us and has 3-10,000 taste buds defining sweet, sour, spicy and bitter.

---

[58] https://www.reference.com/science/many-nerves-bodies-11b1a5bfdb54f2e2

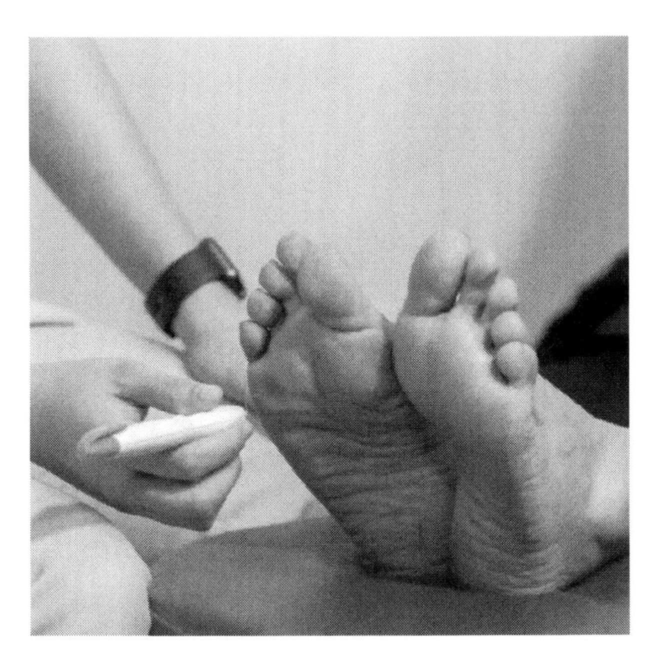

Testing for neuropathy is cheap, effective and reliable. A special tension plastic fibre is used that can apply known pressure. Some with neuropathy would be unable to detect a level of around 10G monofilament.

"Diabetes is associated with increased risk of peripheral neuropathy defined by monofilament insensitivity, but prediabetes and undiagnosed diabetes may be associated with only a modest increase in risk"[59].

[59] Katon JG, Reiber GE, Nelson KM. Peripheral neuropathy defined by monofilament insensitivity and diabetes status. Diabetes Care. 2013 Jun;36(6):1604-6.

Who is most at risk from neuropathy?

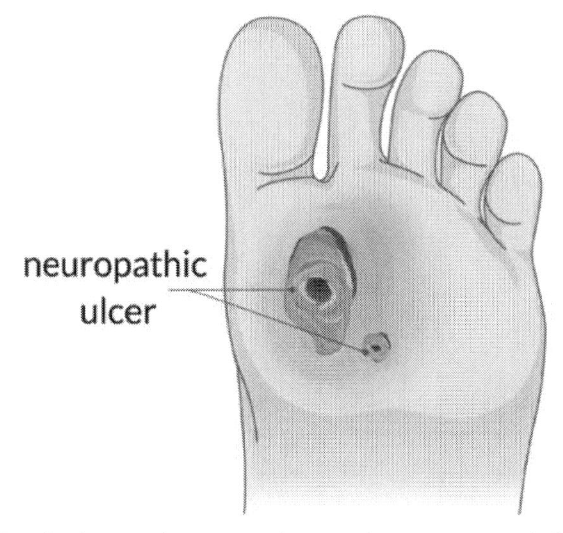

Our body requires an early warning system and the nerves are important for the skin to receive signals as well as the joints.

Ulcers on the sole (plantar surface) of feet pose the greatest concern where illnesses inflict disability which includes the side effect of blindness on top of the inability to feel the foot. When studying medicine in the late seventies I had drummed into me the variable problems of syphilis. Those with this advanced disease caused by a sexually transmitted disease due to Treponema Pallidum, a spiral bacterium. Cases of syphilis in England have increased considerably in recent years: 2019 was the year with the highest number of diagnoses since the 1940s[60].

[60]https://assets.publishing.service.gov.uk/government/uploads/system/uploads/attachment_data/file/956716/Syphilis_Action_Plan_Metrics_2010_to_2019_report.pdf

This infection causes loss of sensation and other sensory functions in the late stages and is called neurogenic syphilis. People exposed can have a high step method of walking called Tabetic gait after the condition *tabes dorsalis* – syphilis to you and me. The walking pattern is created because those infected could not tell where the ground was or where their limbs were when they moved.

There are textbooks that cover the subject of neuropathy in great detail but diseases and disorders that cause loss of sensation include infection at the top of their ranks.

Parasites and bacteria can give rise to nerve damage. The best known condition is cited in the Christian Bible and concerns leprosy. Leper colonies were established to isolate humans from one another as it was thought to be highly infectious. This was not entirely correct.

The infection (mycobacterium leprae), also known as Hansen's disease not only causes loss of cartilage affecting the nose and ears, creating disfigurement but alters the nerve messages and leads skin ulcers which are difficult to heal under the foot. Suffers are forces to walk many miles to seek help in third world countries where health care and education is sub-optimal.

Most readers will be aware of diabetes and this leads to neuropathy only where the disease becomes unstable or ignored so that nerves are affected. Small blood vessels supplying nerves are involved with this deterioration.

Chronic alcoholism and some types of poisoning lead to nerve damage and then there is vitamin deficiency. Vitamin B_{12} is important for nerve development, repair and function. The condition pernicious anaemia is associated with vitamin B_{12} absorption problems in the gut although poor diet can also cause poor nerve function in extreme cases.

Should we put chilblains in hot water?

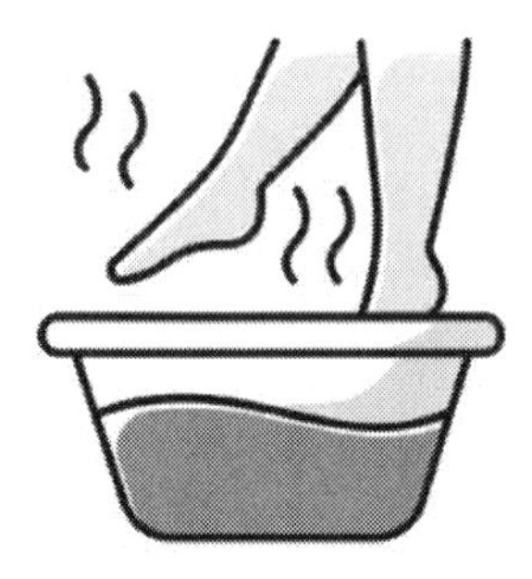

Ever suffered from cold feet - feet that are numbingly cold at that? Cold is unpleasant and the temptation to warm the skin fast is a strong emotional attraction for a quick fix. The answer to the question, *should we use hot water?* may be evident to some.

Chilblains (also called perniosis) are localised inflammatory lesions of the skin associated with cold exposure. Note that pernio-like lesions have been identified as a potential marker for coronavirus disease (COVID-19). Controversy exists at the time of writing as to whether these lesions are a late-stage manifestation of COVID-19 itself. A secondary blood clot tendency created by COVID-19 may be associated with passive activity and the cold.

Chilblains develop acutely. The lesions are either single or multiple and may vary in colour from red to violet and characterised by itching or burning pain. If chilblains do not settle within a few days, blistering and ulceration can even lead to infection. Chilblains are typically located around the skin at the end of fingers and toes, but can affect the nose and ears.

Much of the information in the last paragraph has been simplified [61]. Small vessels in the skin have a unique control on blood flow. Opening and shutting down the cross section (lumen) within blood vessels is called vasodilation and vasoconstriction. Local thermal control of small blood vessels is associated with local sensory nerves and the chemical nitric oxide. Local cooling of the skin can decrease skin blood flow to minimal levels. During menopause, changes in reproductive hormone levels substantially alter thermoregulatory control of skin blood flow. This altered control might contribute to the occurrence of hot flashes.

Medical problems

In type 2 diabetes, the ability of skin blood vessels to dilate is impaired. This impaired vasodilation contributes to the increased risk of heat illness in this patient population during exposure to elevated external temperatures. Raynaud's phenomenon and erythromelalgia relate to disorders of local and/or reflex thermoregulatory control of the skin circulation[62]. *So chilblains are a bit more complex as are the medical names!*

If we intervene with hot water, we cause a sudden interference with the thermoregulation. Heat can damage the skin, but the changes brought about by heat makes the vessel diameter open up too soon. The sudden surge of under oxygenated blood releases unwanted chemicals built-up from when the vessels were narrow when cold. Pain arises because the nerves and tissue release chemicals.

---

[61] Edgerton, CC. Medscape https://reference.medscape.com/viewarticle/850362_3 2 April 2021
62 Charkoudian,N. 2003 Skin blood flow in adult human thermoregulation: how it works, when it does not, and why May;78(5):6,03-12. doi: 10.4065/78.5.603

So, to answer the question - gentle warming is better than dipping feet into warm water, while dry warming with a towel or blanket will create less damage.

One thing we can all relate to is that cold feet can alter our feeling of wellbeing. Be it an inability to sleep or pain on returning back to the warmth. Pity explorers with poor footwear and protection who traipsed the Arctic or Antarctic circles, or those unfortunate prisoners forced to march distances during the time of war and incarceration. And then we have those who suffered Trench Foot in military engagements.

Do you have stand in a trench to get Trench Foot?

Trench foot or immersion foot results from exposure to temperatures of between 0°C to 15°C and the risk increases if the feet are also wet. It occurs when low temperatures restrict blood flow to the affected area. While being exposed as the military would in times of engagement, people can develop symptoms after short periods of exposure[63]. The severity of the injury will depend on the degree of cold, the wetness of the tissue, and how long a person was exposed to these adverse conditions. Trench foot can occur among people that fish for a living and homeless people. Studies have also shown that people of African ethnicity are more likely to develop the condition than Caucasians. The Great War has captured the common appearance of this condition but today we can see hikers exposed on mountain sides as well as those hardened revellers at gigs such as Glastonbury exposed to the cold, mud and wetness after thousands ruin the ground underfoot. Swelling, pain and skin damage arise and in severe cases, fungal infection.

---

[63] https://www.medicalnewstoday.com/articles/145855

Can you really get an elephant foot

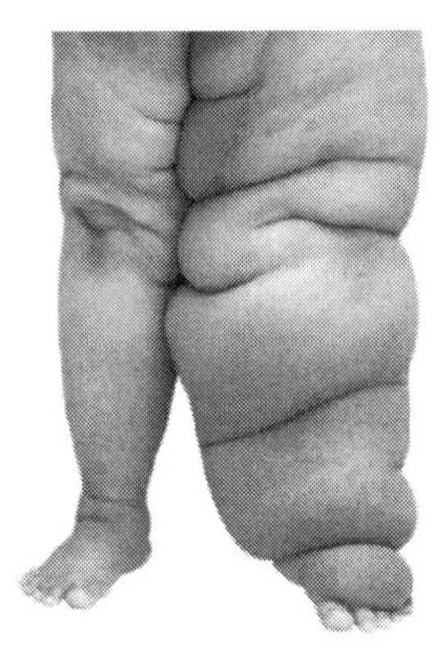

You might have heard of the elephant man - a Victorian oddity called John Merrick, whose head was distorted, but in fact looked nothing like an elephant. He had a condition called *Proteus disease* which affects the development of tissues at a critical stage during foetal development. It just so happens that this condition can affect the foot – distorting it badly. The enlargement is more akin to the enlarged soft pad of this large mammal. Where the leg and foot are affected, another condition is related to infection.

Elephantiasis is a true medical condition. The reason for the gross swelling relates to the drainage vessels known as the lymphatics that no longer work effectively in one or both limbs. The skin thickens and at the top of the leg the genitalia can be affected. While these are the signs, the cause is infective in nature and associated with the tropics. Parasitic worm infections block off the lymphatic vessels and cause the limb to swell creating back pressure. The World Health Organisation estimate that 15 million people suffer from this lymphatic problem[64].

---

[64] https://www.who.int/news-room/fact-sheets/detail/lymphatic-filariasis

The parasite is known as the filariasis worm and we learn that over 120 million in 73 countries suffer from parasitic worms[65]. The thought of worms in our bodies is rather unpleasant. The skin of the foot and limb infected with this parasite becomes thickened like an elephant from which it derives its name with the appearance of an elephant leg. The worms are thread-like and largely associated with *Wucheria bancrofti* in 90% of cases.

A word about lymphatics and veins

Given that the foot is a long way from the heart requires methods to return excess fluid against gravity. We use the veins with small non-returnable valves in the calf to achieve this mechanical ability. Lymphatics support the veins to drain off fluid that if left would pool around the ankles and feet. The lymphatics also help protect against infection with special nests of cells in the groin and armpit. Excessive fluid drains back into the large neck veins for recirculation. We need a constant fluid pressure in the body or our blood pressure would drop.

Travel concerns

Infections due to parasites make fascinating reading and are more of a concern for westerners returning from tropical countries. The idea that only residents of those countries suffer from lymphatic infection is a myth in this day when worldwide travel is possible. Bringing in infection from other countries while on holiday might not be the only problems you might experience. It is worth looking at blood clots under pain in chapter 5.

---

[65] Correll,R An Overview of Elephantiasis. Verywell. Last updated June 2020. https://www.verywellhealth.com/elephantiasis-symptoms-causes-diagnosis-treatment-coping-4174546

5 – Pain

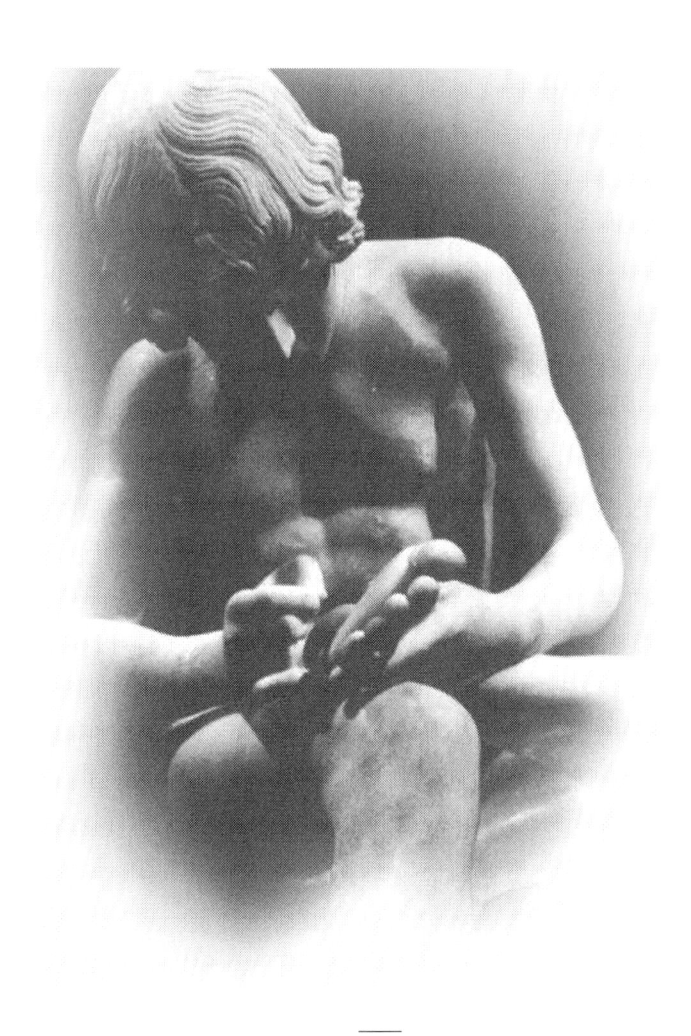

The illustration over the page shows a sculpture known as the *Boy with Thorn*, or *Thorn-Puller* also called *Spinario*. The sculpture was one of the very few Roman bronzes that was never lost to sight. Not surprisingly the statue is often sought after in various materials by podiatrists and is an international symbol for foot pain and the art of podiatric medicine.

Pain is a complex subject, but, for our purposes, most pain is visible, associated with an infection, injury, disease or deformity. It shouldn't surprise the reader that this is the largest chapter in the book.

- Blood clots
- Fractures
- Shin splints
- Arthritis
- Bunions
- Heel spurs
- Footballer's toe
- Dancing en pointe
- Cramp & salt
- Metatarsalgia
- Morton's neuroma
- Ingrown toe nail

Can you really get a blood clot from flying?

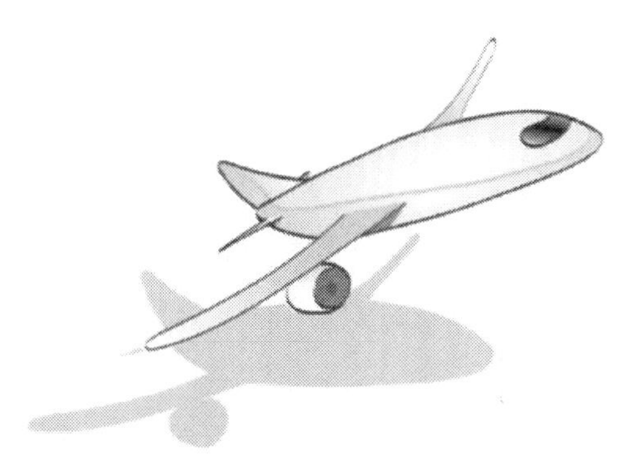

We all enjoy going abroad as long haul flights have become popular. So is the blood clot associated with flying just a myth? We know from experience prolonged bed rest after a hospital intervention poses a high risk. The lack of movement of muscles responsible for moving blood back through the heart to energise with fresh oxygen is a factor. Flights with limited movement in squashed seats and too much alcohol add to these risks. Other risks include:-

- personal or family history of blood clots
- being 40 or older
- smoking cigarettes
- being overweight
- medication such as the birth control pill or HRT
- having had a surgical procedure or immobilised injury
- cancer treatment
- pregnancy

Clots can be life threatening. Always seek medical advice before travelling if you fit the profile.

Do we only have foot fractures at certain times of the year?

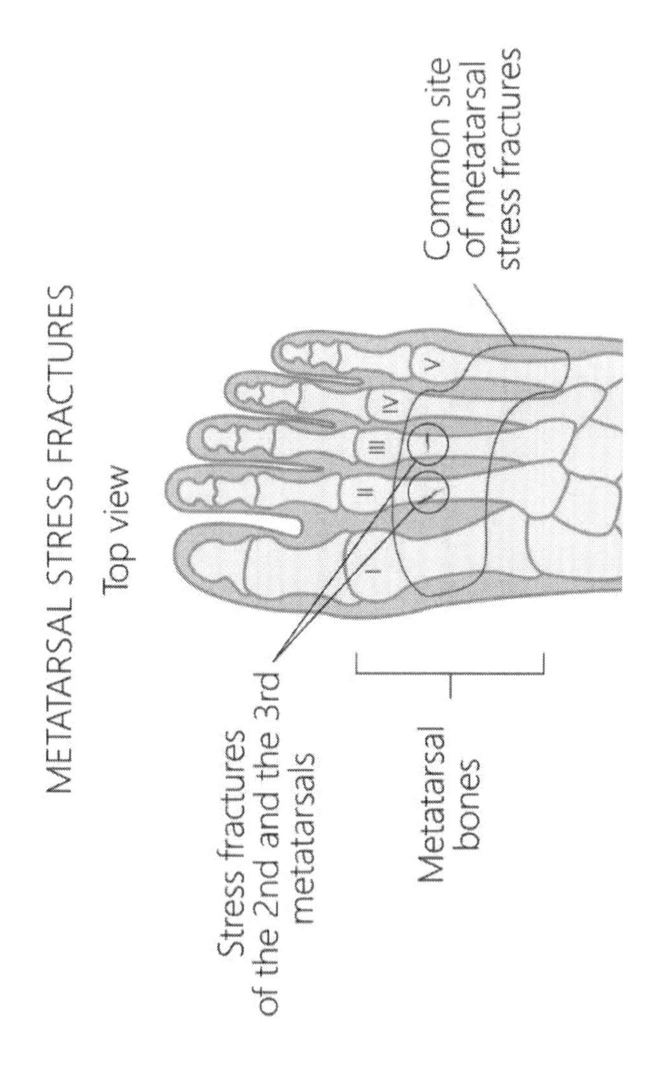

March or stress fracture

Fractures or breaks in feet are not constrained by weather or seasons. Many fractures occur in dry conditions at any time of the year and in the home. The term 'march fracture' was associated with soldiers and the practice of 'square bashing'. The constant stamping of feet would set up tiny stressors in the outer layer (cortex), especially in the longer metatarsal bones. The second metatarsal was particularly exposed because it is regarded as longer. Stress fractures, unlike full breaks, will heal in time but require rest. The metatarsal is prone over other bones as it acts as a lever during activity, meaning you don't have to be a soldier to sustain a stress fracture.

Why are stress fractures missed?

The diagram on the opposite page shows the general area where metatarsal fractures occur. The neck of the 2nd and 3rd bones shown, suggest a crack. X-rays fail to show up small changes early on and can be missed.

Once healing commences, the resultant process associated with the crack is visible on x-ray. The cortex swells and new bone is laid down. This may take 2-3 weeks and a repeat x-ray is needed to reveal the crack that an earlier x-ray did not. Stress fractures usually heal without intervention. Ongoing pain should be investigated and an open mind retained. Failed healing can be confused with a rare bone cancer.

Other fractures found in the foot

Sporting activities can cause fractures anywhere in the foot. Tendons are strong as are their attachments, but sudden twisting forces can create significant damage. These problems do not settle without intervention.

If the tendon breaks or causes a chunk of bone to pull out (avulsion) then pain will become chronic.

The worst fractures are those where the bone is separated into pieces or pushed into joints such as in road traffic accidents. Fractures through joints can damage growing cartilage. If this happens in the child with an immature, undeveloped foot, permanent damage is sustained. Small bones of the midfoot occasionally have cracks and elude immediate x-ray diagnosis.

It is rare for hospital accident departments to fix toe fractures and most doctors just tape toes together as a 'buddy'. The downside to this is they become sweaty, inflamed or even create a sensitivity to the dressing. Fractures of this type tend to heal from 4-8 weeks unless there is more than a crack or stress line. Not all fractures require a leg or foot cast. A stiff soled shoe works well as long as swelling is allowed.

Is the ankle part of the foot?

The ankle links the foot with the lower leg bones through the steering wheel called the talus. This was discussed in the first chapter. It is worth bearing in mind that the foot is controlled by tendons, blood vessels and nerves that connect through the ankle to the foot. Injury and fractures from the ankle to the hip can influence pain in the foot. Referred pain is an expression where pain is located further-a-field than the site of the original injury. This paradox compounds the difficulty with identifying some pain problems which have no rhyme or reason being in the foot. The best known referred sign in the foot is a slipped lumbar disc where the big toe is numb due to nerve interference. A drop foot can be associated with a nerve being associated with a fracture of the outer leg bone (fibula) below the knee.

Why is leg pain called a shin splint?

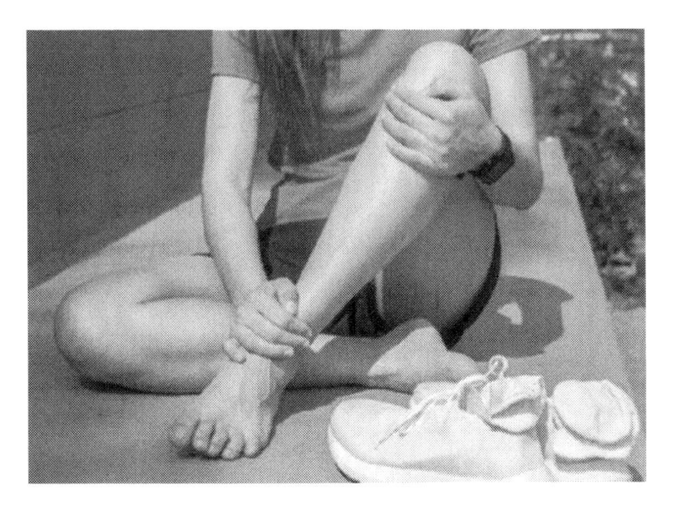

This is a common term known amongst runners and often called *runners' shin splints*. If you are into sports then you may be familiar with this condition. The increased passion for running brought this condition to the fore in the eighties, although of course it would have affected ancient armies forced to march toward their antagonists seeking battle. Of course the army 'sawbones' at the time might have sought unconventional remedies with potentially fatal consequences. Unfortunately such conditions were not recorded in detail. *Fact or fiction* –shin splints while not a 20th or 21st century feature, affects, hardy walkers and there is no reason to assume it did not affect foot soldiers from bygone years. The leg bone or tibia has a flat inner surface we know as the shin. Muscles run off either side of this surface and feed onto the foot via tendons. Muscle is attached via fibres to the bone through a membrane called the periosteum which is supplied by blood on the outside of the bone.

Any tissue with blood can become inflamed if irritated and can lead to a haematoma along the shin. This means that a clump of blood has formed. The activity of slamming the foot down on the ground builds up shock waves that will project back up the tibia. This repetitive nature sets up stress and this can lead to small fractures in the bone or tears that damage the periosteum. Swelling and inflammation are the ingredients for discomfort. A searing hot pain along the shin leads to the suspicion of an *overuse syndrome*.

Chronic pain

Chronic shin splints may have uneven bumps from repeated inflammation making the normal smooth sensation lumpy. Haematomas can change to bone in some cases adding to the rough sensation on examination. Treatment is rest and activity paced with shorter strides. Shock absorbing shoes and inlays (orthoses) are of enormous help. The condition will affect any age or gender and can be reversed. Where shin splints appear to worsen, or the leg or foot swells, then *compartment syndrome* must be considered. Although rare, this can be an emergency. Fluid builds up which compresses on blood vessels and nerves affecting the flow of blood to the lower limb. Death of muscle and skin lead to that horrific scene of gangrene.

Is gangrene - green?

Well John Hopkins provides the answer. Gangrene often turns the affected skin a greenish-black color. However, the word gangrene is not related to the color green, but to the condition itself. It comes from Greek and Latin words for a gnawing sore or decayed tissue[66].

---

[66]https://www.hopkinsmedicine.org/health/conditions-and-diseases/gangrene

Is damage inside the foot called arthritis?

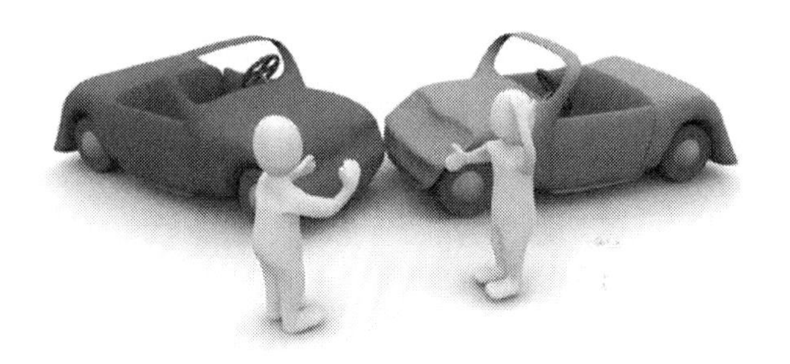

When it comes to risk from failure to act after foot injuries, then the consequences, while not life-threatening, can lead to a form of disability that affects the quality of life.

The road traffic accident is a good example. If the body is at risk from bleeding out, or the heart stops, or the brain is damaged, the lower limb and foot may be the least of the concerns of the emergency services unless it is visibly damaged and at risk from – yes you guessed it – gangrene.

If you zip back to my opening chapter on delayed effect and timeline resulting from injury, we see foot pain can arise later on. We need to go inside the joint to consider the effects. Just as cars age and breakdown, so does our body.

Do I have arthritis?

There are a few medical words that have become incorrectly applied to pain and joints. *"My doctor says I have arthritis,"* is just as likely to be a working diagnosis that placates the average patient because it is a label. Labels are unhelpful, and when wrongly applied mislead the patient, delaying the real mystery behind the problem. Arthritis is a medical condition sure enough, but it is very specific. Arthritis and inflammation go together but there are many causes. As we age we do lose cartilage as it thins and sometimes two bone ends will grate on each other. In medical parlance we suggest this sounds like crunching 'celery'. There is a normal ageing process of degeneration rather than the disease called arthritis; we call this physiological *wear and tear*. The word arthrosis is more useful. While non-specific it implies a condition of the joint with deterioration. Stiffness may arise and cause pain, but it may be put down to this wear and tear rather than a medical entity like osteoarthritis or rheumatoid arthritis. Wear and tear arthrosis in feet includes the big toe which then stiffens and causes pain, or midfoot arthrosis with the addition of bone formation.

Osteoarthritis (OA) in feet is not as prolific as in the hands where the finger joints are targeted. The big joints such as the hip, knee and ankle are common to OA. This condition affects older people, over 45 as a broad guide and relates to defective cartilage quality superimposed by overuse, injury and weight gain. To add confusion symptoms, which include stiffness, are shared by other forms of arthrosis.

Rheumatoid arthritis is part of an autoimmune disorder where feet are commonly affected. This can afflict children and used to be called Still's disease but now known as juvenile chronic arthritis.

Deformity can arise leaving toes out of alignment and some patients are bedridden. Modern drug therapy relies less on steroids now than is the past and the most significant deformities are arrested earlier than they were quarter of a century ago. Arthritis is often combined with the term arthrosis, a condition of the joints where specific conditions are described. Three other lesser known, but no less painful conditions involving the foot include gouty arthritis, which affects the big toe, and **ankylosing spondylosis** that can affect the heel as well as the spine. **Gout** (illustrated) is associated with rich foods containing purines. Faulty metabolism causes uric acid build up. **Psoriatic arthritis** affects 7% of those with skin psoriasis and whittles away metatarsal ends into points.

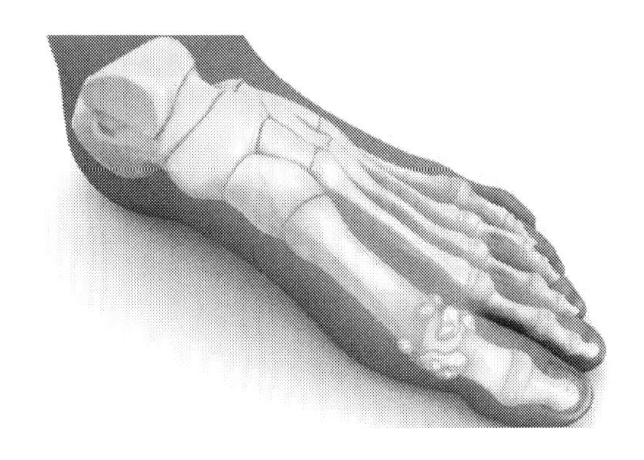

Does a blood test show up gout in my toe?

A blood test is often used to show increased levels of monosodium urate. The fact is that we can obtain false readings. Put simply, the blood test may be inaccurate. The question you might ask is why is this test not always reliable? The diagnostic rule relies heavily on the presence of increased serum urate blood concentration which often arises in normal during a gout flare due to increased kidney waste removal (excretion) during the acute phase of the condition. The levels of urate should be rechecked 2–4 weeks after the flare resolves. The condition affects five times as many men as women in the general population, and the test is not sufficient to make a diagnosis of gout in the absence of symptoms[67]. A conclusive diagnosis may require a sample of joint fluid to highlight the crystals. Within the joint chronic crystallisation takes on the appearance of the content of crushed almonds.

Are x-rays required for pain?

X-rays are valuable and patients feel they must have one or the doctor has failed. This common imaging technique shows deformity, dislocation, bone thickness, reduced joint spaces, and many affectations with medical diseases or injury. Not every aspect of damage can be decided from an x-ray because the image can only provide collaborative information. Cartilage is not visible on images (see page 69). It is not until we go inside the joint that we see the effects of cartilage damage. We can conclude that x-rays do not provide an accurate picture of inside the joint.

Are bunions arthritis?

True or false? *If you have hallux valgus, will you have degeneration in the toe?* But this is not necessarily due to arthritis. For every hallux valgus I have corrected, I would estimate 70% have some form of cartilage damage. In an Austrian study, 73% of 265 joints (196 patients) had erosions[68], being cartilage defects (p.143).

---

[67] Dalbeth, N, Gosling,AL, Gaffo,A. Abhishek A. Lancet 2021; 397: 1843–55 March 30, 2021 https://doi.org/10.1016/ S0140-6736(21)00569-9

[68] Bock, P, Kristen, KH, Kroner, A, Engel A,. Hallux valgus and cartilage degeneration in the first metatarsophalangeal joint. JBJS. 86-B(5):669-673

The researchers followed 79% of their patients for two years. The moral of this tale makes clear that only by following patients for any length can we work out the *timeline effect* applied to treatment[69]. The illustration below was taken from one of my own patients where the arrows reveal cartilage erosions common in hallux valgus. The patient depicted in the picture below could expect stiffness after surgery but this would not necessarily affect recovery except in rare cases. Research has confirmed that patients do well.

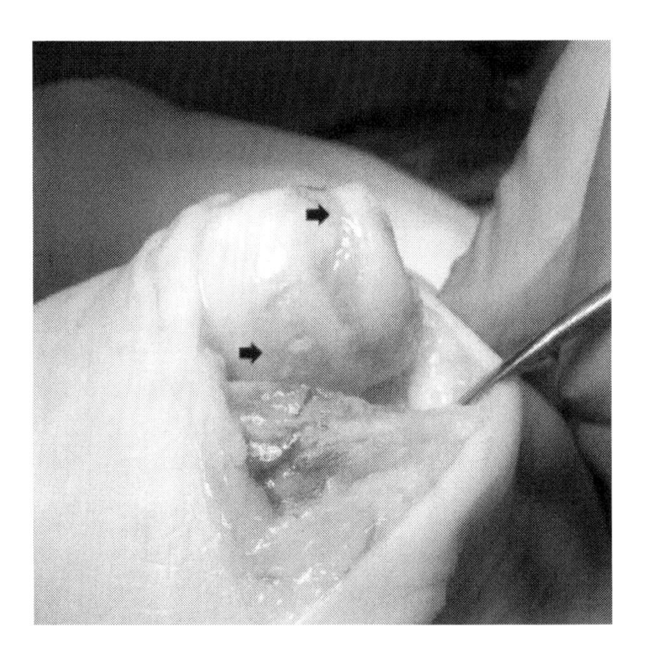

[69] Jastifer, JR, Coughlin, MJ, Doty, JF, Stevens, FR, Hirose, C, Kemp, TJ. Osteochondral lesions in surgical treatment of hallux valgus. Am. Orth. Foot & Ankle Soc. 2014, 35(7):643-649

Does cartilage damage make a difference to your treatment?

The extent of joint damage observed at surgery does not always agree with the severity of the deformity. However, as the deformity increases, the number of defects increases. The loss of the lubrication leads to cartilage drying? We cannot predict the incident of erosions before surgery without more expensive imaging methods. We can say that it is more likely than not that patients with pain associated with the first toe joint will have erosions. Joint-related research must continue to look for more evidence. We need high study numbers because current research tends to use lower numbers than in older research. Ethical consideration and tighter criteria have limited active cohort participation.

Ethics and research

The word *ethics* crops up in all human research and must be approved by an authority of experts to comply with safety in mind, as well as having a purpose that will benefit science. Following the Nazi regime (1933-45) and in particular the Holocaust, experiments were conducted in inhumane conditions and without safeguard for the subjects dignity or their value of life. International laws were passed to govern all aspects of scientific experimentation and all pharmacy products must follow a similar code. This subject is extensive and can only be glossed over here and yet it is important. We will meet more ethical considerations under the chapter on Fables with the 'silicone experiment'.

Are spurs the cause of heel pain?

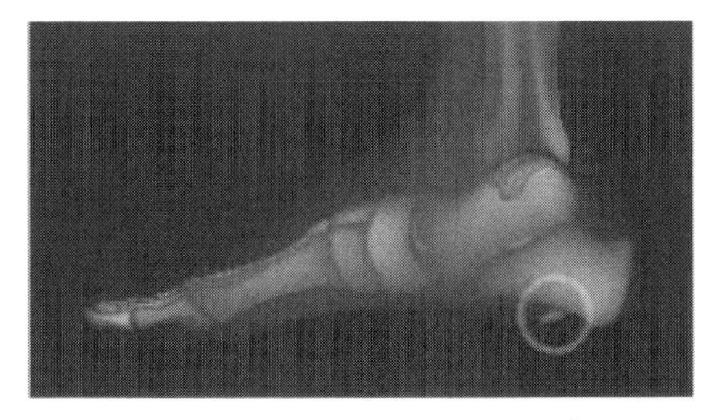

Nothing has been so maligned than the heel spur in causing heel pain. Professionals offering musculoskeletal (MSK) skills have to consider a range of potential causes of heel discomfort but the spur is often the first diagnosis given. Radiologists, the doctors who read x-rays and provide a diagnosis, believe a positive spur is conclusive. However, there is lack of clarity amongst professionals attributing a spur to heel pain. Patients presented with a diagnosis of plantar fasciitis[70] and had x-rays compared to those taken at the same hospital with ankle sprain. Johal and Milner believed there to be a correlation between the spur and plantar fasciitis[71], a condition affecting the band of tissue from heel to toe, but went on to make the statement in their discussion, "*Whilst acknowledging that the true association between plantar fasciitis and calcaneal spur formation may have been weaker than our data suggests if some of the comparison subjects had in fact suffered from plantar fasciitis but did not have a calcaneal spur, we must also recognise that two patients with a diagnosis of plantar fasciitis did not have spurs, thus making accurate prediction difficult.*"

---

[70] PF or plantar fasciopathy is now considered fasciopathy or fasciosis

[71] Johal, KS, Milner SA Plantar Fasciitis and the calcaneal spur: Fact or fiction? Foot and Ankle Surgery 2011, 18;39-41

Johal and Miller's study was small. Other researchers' views are unclear. Kirkpatrick looked at the anatomy closely and felt the idea of the fascia being involved alone with heel pain still required more investigation[72].

Single case reports can reveal how an extremely large spur appeared in a young male without chronic disease responded without surgery. All pain subsided and he regained full function of his foot. This case questions the association between the size of the heel spur and plantar fasciitis symptoms. The problem is not associated with plantar fasciitis[73]. In a study of 1335 patients, x-rays were reviewed to compare age with the spur. There was a significant correlation between older patients where the spur increased in size[74].

Location of spur and plantar fascia

There is evidence to suggest that spur and fascia are not entirely related but many authors conclude that spur presence and fascia occur together. This does not present the whole picture because it is a fact that you can have a spur and no pain. The projecting spur is a ledge of bone that goes all the way across the heel bone. The fascial band sits below the so-called spur and so does not pull on the heel bone (calcaneus). The fascial band does not pull the spur out like a piece of stretching chewing gum. The main heel bone develops around 6-8 years.

---

[72] Kirkpatrick J, Yassaie O, Mirjalili SA. The plantar calcaneal spur: a review of anatomy, histology, etiology and key associations. *J Anat.* 2017;230(6):743-751. doi:10.1111/joa.12607

[73] Alatassi,R Alajlan,,A, Almalki,T. Bizarre calcaneal spur: A case report, International Journal of Surgery Case Reports, 2018, 49:37-39,

[74] Beytemür O, Öncü M. The age dependent change in the incidence of calcaneal spur. *Acta Orthop Traumatol Turc.* 2018;52(5):367-371. doi:10.1016/j.aott.2018.06.013

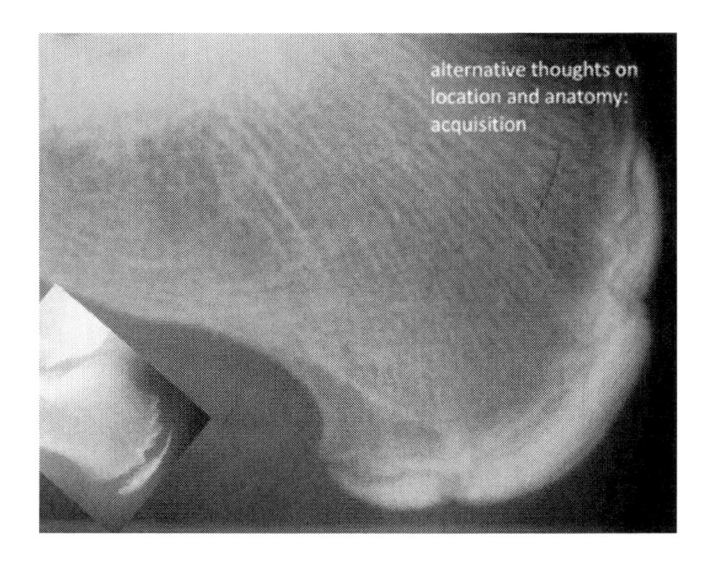

A smaller part of the heel bone increases in size and unites with the main bone at 12-14 years. The gap is evident from the x-ray (shown above) in the juvenile, where the bones have not united. The ledge or spur in its' primacy and youngsters tend not to suffer from plantar fasciitis.

Moral of the tale

Yes, you can have heel pain with a so-called spur, but it does not relate to pulling of the band as muscles may be involved. The moral of this tale to date is that surgery is not necessary for almost all cases because conservative care can minimise such as approach. Argument remain over the spur and fasciitis but the gap is closing.

Do you have to join the police to get policeman's heel?

For some strange reason occupational names stick and suggest that only certain groups suffer from a particular condition. Policeman's heel in fact was put down to pain from a swelling called a bursa. A bursa is a sac of fluid as discussed earlier.

Today this has morphed into a wider range of syndromes that really means any condition affecting the contact surface of the heel. The bursa sits under the main heel bone but so often it is the plantar fascial fibres that run from toes to heel that are inflamed around the heel. Swelling of the heel pad is a give-away sign.

By now we should be aware of overuse and repetitive strains. Plantar fasciitis is common in all walks of life following episodes of activity, affecting one or both feet. Doubtless the condition would once have been associated with the spur which is no longer considered relevant as a common condition. The spur still remains a way to explain away heel pain, and patients are accepting of this as a fact.

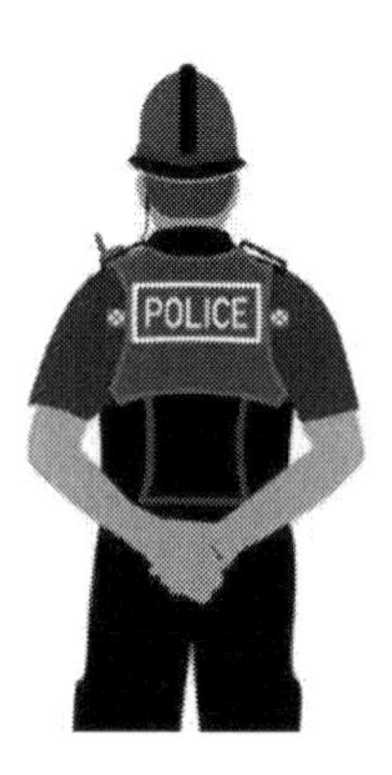

Footballer's (soccer's) toe

Another condition attributed to an occupation affects the big toe. In fact this is more often called *Turf Toe*.

The foot and toe is stubbed and impacts against soft or hard ground causing damage to the joint. Although the ball is usually kicked from the side of the foot, a direct kick from the end of the toe is more significant. Pain and swelling in the first toe joints can lead to long standing injury. It is worth going back to cartilage damage to read about the same problem, only this condition does not relate to hallux valgus but a condition called rigid toe or hallux rigidus.

The toe slowly stiffens, reduces the range of movement which in turn affects the way the foot works with the lower limb. Men probably suffer more than women based on clinical presentation. Active people are at greater risk from sports, hobbies and occupations exposed to toe stubbing, which includes the bedroom! The increased awareness of health and safety at work, together with the use of safety footwear, has helped minimise foot injuries.

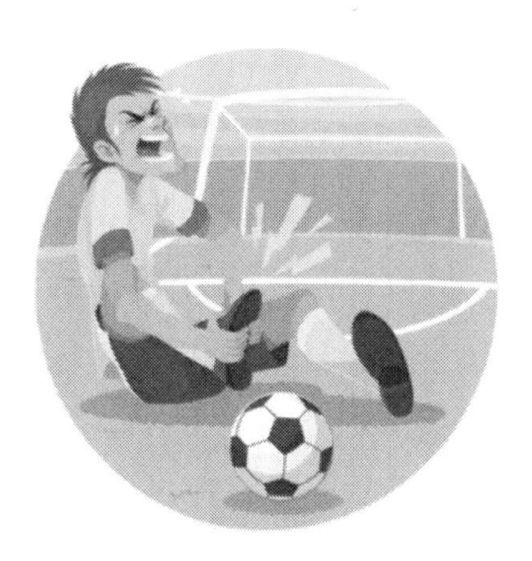

Are black toenails dangerous?

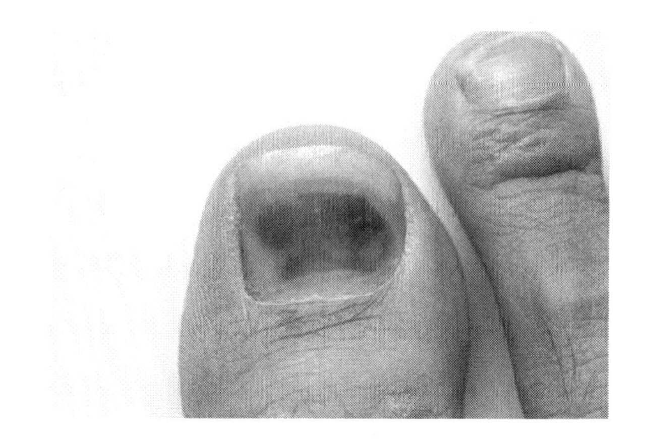

Anyone can sustain a black toe injury and it looks pretty ugly after the initial pain goes. Having met the word haematoma earlier. Blood remains under the nail when it is not released and this discolours the nail. It goes without saying that footballers can experience nail damage with turf toe.

The idea that toes go black is often associated with dry gangrene, but toe nails may also go black in part or whole because the skin forming the nail bed has a pigmented lesion called a melanoma.

If the toe has been injured and bleeds underneath, the darkness disappears in time and grows forward as the nail grows. However, the size and shape of the dark colour can vary from a pool of dark to streaks and these require urgent referral. Malignant melanoma are highly dangerous if left. If dealing with a GP receptionist you must say you have a problem on which you need an urgent opinion using the word 'malignant'. Even if it turns out to be a false alarm it is never a waste of time to have it checked. Receptionists should not question the word malignancy – but don't abuse this suggestion.

Should Dancers go en Pointe!

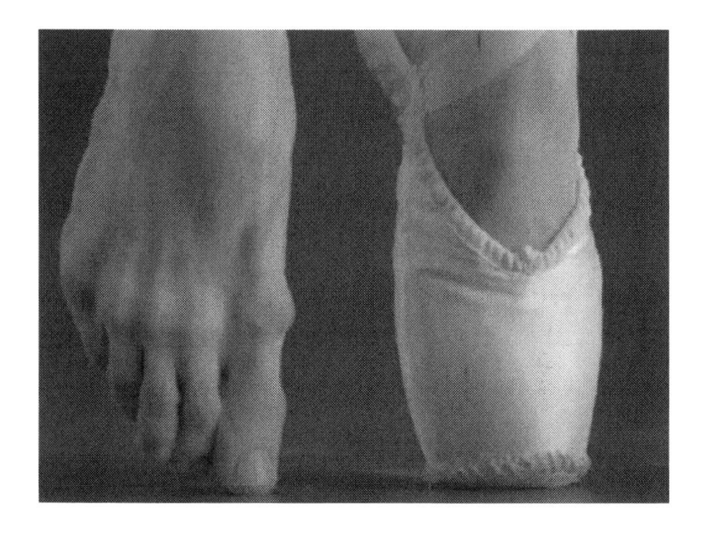

No one can remain unaffected by the beautiful spectacle dancers put on. We pick up the Chinese story around the beautiful lotus foot position. The foot balances on the toes. But what of the damage? Look at any popular chick flicks covering dancing. Some hunk will be on hand to nurse blisters and sprains. Pointe dancing, that is dancing on the extreme ends of the toes with the aid of a toe shoe, as performed by the advanced female ballet dancer, causes unnatural loading of the foot[75]. Conditions such as skin blisters, callus, soft tissue damage and degenerative joint damage can arise. To determine the effectiveness of a ballet shoe, the authors measured the normal pressure distribution on the foot en pointe.

[75] R. G. Torba and D. A. Rice, "Pressure analysis of the ballet foot while en pointe," *Biomedical Engineering Conference, 1993., Proceedings of the Twelfth Southern*, New Orleans, LA, USA, 1993, pp. 48-50.doi: 10.1109/SBEC.1993.247350

Sampling the entire forefoot in the toebox of a pointe shoe showed that pressures arise over the bony prominences and the ends of the toes.

The strains on the forefoot account for about 80% of the total force bearing down on the foot. The skin takes up the remaining energy.

The great toe receives considerable body force, not just going onto 'point' but due to constant impact. The square toebox helps, but the foot takes a battering. Inside these joints, a slow process emerges over time leaving a dancer with a high chance of arthropathy later in life as cartilage does not repair. The rule comes from a guideline about not going onto the toes until 12 years of age[76] . This is considered appropriate as growth centres (plates) are easily injured earlier than this age group. The foot however tends not to mature until 14-16 in girls and 15-17 in boys.

According to the International Association of Dance Medicine & Science, the type of dance is important, not the age. In the case of girls, 12 is not the maturation age.

Later life and timeline

Moving into adulthood, the effects of impact trauma to the great toe are all too easy to see. Small bleeds lead to scar attachment, while tears in the cartilage may not cause pain, new bone formation develops and this affects available movement. If this happens at the great toe, the midfoot and hindfoot, each joint will bear the pain and pleasure of this specialised pastime. It is for the dedicated alone to survive the rigours and effects of dancing as in most high levels sports. Later on in life payback arises.

---

[76] Guidelines for initiating Pointe training J. Dance Medicine & Science 13,(3)90-92

Do we get foot cramps because of a lack of salt?

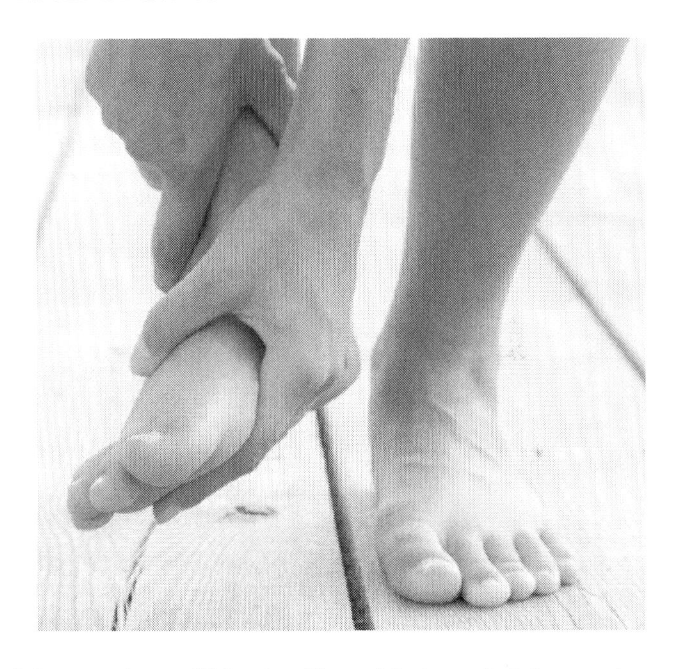

Most readers will be familiar with the painful sensation of cramps. While affecting our legs or thighs, what about our feet? One myth to quell cramp was to eat a banana because this had potassium, a significant body salt. The subject of cramp is by no means a small topic so let us address the key elements.

There are medical reasons for cramping and stomach cramps that fall into this bundle of concerns and include monthly menstruation, but there is no record for the affected feet. However, sexual intercourse can set off foot cramps, which is a procreational exercise.

A cramp is an involuntary forceful muscle contraction that takes a while to relax. The pain from cramp is uncomfortable and feels like an 'intense gripping' sensation. When the muscle settles and eases a dull ache is often left behind. You might have to cease activity if the muscle keeps cramping and you may wake up the next day with the muscle feeling tender, but you should be able to function well.

Foot cramp

The two areas likely to cause painful cramps are in the small muscles of the feet. If you want to be more academic, the inside arch has a muscle called the *abductor hallucis*, which attaches to the base of the big toe. The other group of seven small muscles that go into spasm are called the *interossei* and lie between the metatarsals. When these fire off, as I like to call it – in other words - contract, the pain is pretty horrible. Brett Sears [77] agrees with these observations when he describes the cramping scenario that can occur at night or in bed and wake you up with pain. The trouble is that cramps can occur at any time, in hot and cold. So what about this salt argument?

Athletes had their blood levels measured based on their loss of water in sweat and hence loss of salt. The findings showed there was little difference between those who suffered cramp and those that didn't. Next, Miller[78] tried to see if cramps could be produced by using an electric current in brave volunteers. It turns out that the scientific community has found no isolated cause for sudden eruptions of cramp.

---

[77] https://www.verywellhealth.com/brett-sears-2695988

[78] Miller, KC, Harsen, JD, Long, BC Prophylactic Stretching Does Not Reduce Cramp Susceptibility. School of Rehabilitation and Medical Sciences, Central Michigan University. Accepted 5 August 2017

What can you do about cramping?

Well, any podiatrist will tell you to ensure that your footwear fits and is not tight across the front of the foot – the widest part. A curious finding that you might consider anecdotal arises from the smaller interossei mentioned before going onto spasm, compressing an important digital nerve to be discussed in the next section. Brought on by tight cycling shoe gear, I paid a heavy price because the nerve was squashed in my narrow shoe.

Returning to Miller's work, he found that stretching did not prevent cramps in his 15 volunteers. He hypothesises that nerve innervation is more likely to be the culprit than dehydration.

Is there a solution?

When it comes to my own experience, I stretch out the cramped spasm aggressively. First, the toe muscles are flexed and extended manually by stretching out the toe tendons and their muscles by hand.

Secondly, where the arch spasms, I stand and push down on the ball of my big toe (metatarsal head). By elongating the foot, the arch is stretched, aiding the muscle fibres. Forced stretching can help the immediate discomfort, but cramps can return. Again, hot or cold makes little difference, but I use bed socks if my feet are too cold and believe this helps. Of course, more severe forms of cramp exist, but in the case of the myth surrounding salt causing an isolated foot cramp, this appears more fiction than fact in its milder form.

Does metatarsalgia affect metatarsals?

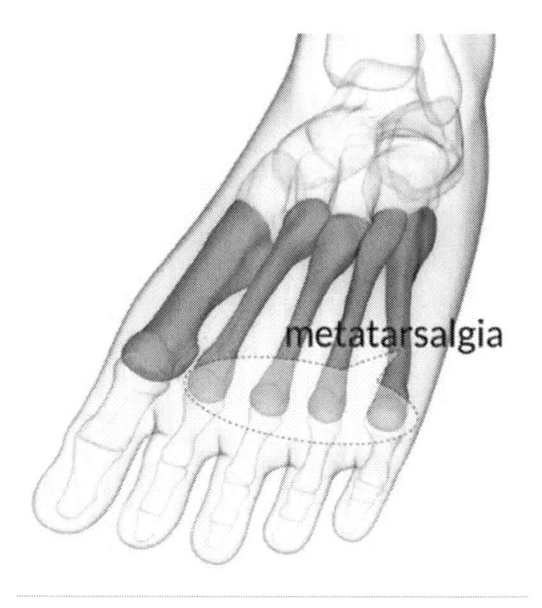

A broad term

Metatarsalgia is a broad term for pain that affects the front – ball of the foot (see outline above). The question many ask, are the metatarsals affected? Most medical terms come from Latin, while some are Greek, affording medicine the status of both a religion and a new language.

Today all medical students learn this language, one with mixed ancient words alongside their mother tongue.

'...algia' is derived from the Greek algos meaning pain. Metatarsal is the long foot bone and one of five. We have met words like talus, then there is the tibia which in Latin means *shinbone* but also *pipe* and *flute*. Seemingly bones had a function like the slim fibula or broach bone. The point being made is that medical terminology is vast and originates from the ancient Hellenistic world. We met fractures associated with the curious name March fracture. This is one cause of pain in the ball of the foot and accompanied by swelling. It is easy to diagnose and resolves satisfactorily.

Non-words for medical conditions

Metatarsalgia, like rheumatism is a non-word. We have met another non-word, arthritis, when it is not the disease but a collection of conditions bearing similar signs. Rheumatism actually means inflammation of muscles and joints but it is non-specific and that is what is meant by a non-word, not that it has no meaning.

The commonest causes of metatarsalgia include fracture, joint inflammation called synovitis, a cartilage condition in the adolescent, called osteochondrosis. Skin conditions such as warts and corns, foreign bodies like animal hair must be excluded, but will add to foot pain. The bruised fat pad and swelling caused by a bursa (shown) is not uncommon.

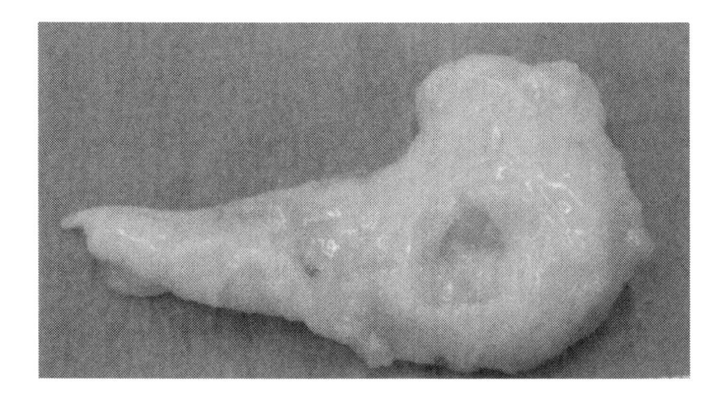

Just to make life difficult we have the medical arthritic conditions such as psoriatic and rheumatoid arthritis; all these forms of arthritis affect the metatarsal region of the foot. Synovitis is caused by a number of conditions and medical disease must be ruled out and covers conditions from Crohn's disease, affecting the bowel, to an overuse injury of the metatarsal-toe joint(s).

The bursa is chronic degenerative soft tissue which relies on adaption of inflammatory cells. Pressure caused by injury, inflammatory arthritis and entry from foreign particles can create this formation in the foot, often the sole. A rigid first toe is one of the most common reasons for pressure and pain under the ball of the foot.

Bone and cartilage growth problems

One of the least common problems associated with metatarsalgia is a condition that causes a disturbance to the growth of the 2nd and sometimes 3rd metatarsal head development – Freiberg's disease. This is not a disease and was first called Freiberg's infraction. It is an adolescent condition and named after Alfred (Henry) Freiberg in 1914[79]. Now this all might sound interesting but Freiberg, an orthopaedic surgeon, published his findings after six women presented with pain in their forefoot, in an obstetrics and gynaecology journal!

Of more interest, this condition may be missed as asymptomatic and appear later in adulthood but arising initially, in adolescence. Metatarsalgia does not affect the metatarsals alone but joints, soft tissue and skin. We now need to look at the most common metatarsal pain associated with a nerve – Morton's neuroma.

[79] https://emedicine.medscape.com/article/1236085-overview#showall

Why is a nerve pain called Morton's Neuroma

Of all the metatarsalgia pains, an unpleasant sensation is experienced as an electric shock toward the toes when compressed. It can be a very confusing set of symptoms from cramping to shooting, aching and throbbing. It is possible to experience hot burning sensations as well as numbness. Morton's neuroma or plantar digital neuritis is also part of the metatarsalgia family.

Who's name was it really?

Durlacher wrote a book in 1845 and covered neuroma[80] describing the condition;

> "A kind of neuralgia seated between the toes, but which fortunately is not very common...the patient complains of pain between two of the toes, generally the second and third, they can seldom tell...it is increased when the toes are pressed together."

Thomas G Morton described the location for the neuroma as the 3rd interspace and this was stretched to include the 2nd interspace, probably more by accident than design. Morton, a surgeon, would also have had a wider audience than Durlacher and expanded his fame through lectures. Communication methods did not have the benefit of the internet.

---

[80] Durlacher, L A treatise on corns, bunions, the diseases of the nail: and the general management of the feet. London: Simpkin, Marshall & Co 1845

Is a neuroma a tumour?

Fact – the nerve thickens but is not a tumour as suggested by the suffix, the end part (*-oma)* of the word. Originally from Greek origins, tumour means swelling and can be many times the normal size because of scar tissue. The problem, alluded to earlier, is the fact that as Durlacher stated, *"patients ...can seldom tell..."* and thus symptoms are indeed confusing because pains can mimic other metatarsalgic conditions. Of the most easily missed are joint inflammation (synovitis) and a torn ligament around the under surface of the toe (metatarso-phalangeal) joint.

Neuroma and the sexes

If we accept that some diseases are genetic, we see a unique set of rules. The haemophilia gene is carried by females but only affects men. However, when it comes to conditions like the bunion and Morton's neuroma, we say that it affects women more than men. This fact is true –6:2 female : male (65 cases) where the incidence in gender is biased toward females[81].

Footwear influence

While footwear causes neuroma problems, many complain of muscle spasm of the small foot muscles (interossei and lumbricals). Most conditions in the foot affect both gender groups. They are not equal because of such as footwear. I will get on to high heels a little later on.

[81] Tollafield D R 2016 National Database Survey Neuroma Surgery. WWW.PASCOM-10

Can Toe Shape Cause Morton's neuroma?

My obsession with Morton's neuroma came from the fact that I actually had the condition and required treatment. This places me at an advantage as a patient and a clinician. You can read more in my book *Podiatrist Turned Patient*[82] - you will have to forgive me for being a bit academic about the subject.

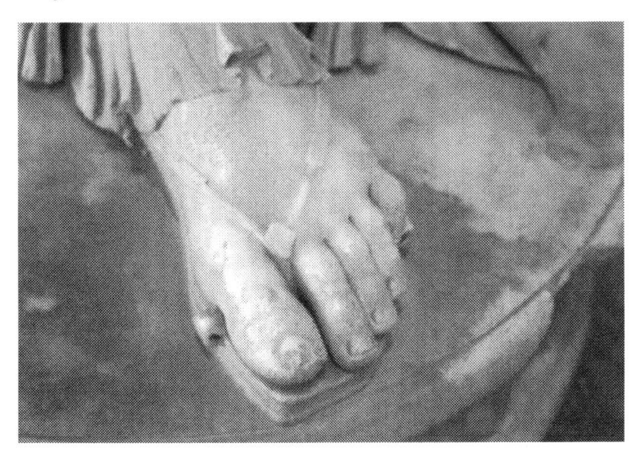

Ancient Statues

Statues from the ancient world can reflect different shapes of feet. There is nothing more curious than observing different toe lengths. The Egyptians suggest a second toe similar in length to the first, while the Greek foot represented their populace with a long second toe.

---

[82] Tollafield, DR, Morton's Neuroma. Podiatrist Turned Patient: My own journey. Busypencilcase Communications 2018. Amazon books. E-book & paperback

Dudley Morton, (no relation of Thomas G Morton) in 1927 was interested in the genealogy of the first toe and considered the Greek foot predominated Morton's neuroma. Jump repeated the study with 184 patients that looked back over old records (retrospective) and formed two groups. In 133 cases taken from his Group A, patients were selected as a control. Twenty per cent (20%) had Greek foot and without symptoms.

When considering Group B, of the group with foot pain and suspected neuroma, 63% had symptoms in the Greek foot, and 37% had symptoms in the Egyptian foot type. While the association suggests a greater chance of having a neuroma in the Greek foot, there has been no conclusive proof. I decided to test this theory out on my own patients.

Testing the theory

The metatarsal length was assessed against the presence of a neuroma. Laboratory reports were reviewed and compared with available x-rays[83]. Two radiographers looked at the x-rays. Results showed that most presented with the Greek foot style and associated with neuroma (68.6%). This smaller sample agreed with Jump. The digital shape of the Greek foot appears to have a higher risk of neuroma than the Egyptian toe length. This was an audit rather than a controlled piece of clinical research and a larger study would be of interest.

Neuroma of the metatarsals creates a wide range of symptoms that can radiate into the hindfoot. Sensations can be painful, affect normal walking, produce shooting, burning and numb type pain. More information is available on this condition[84]

[83] Tollafield & Mehr. Unpublished internal audit 2017

[84] https://consultingfootpain.co.uk

Myths about ingrown toe nails

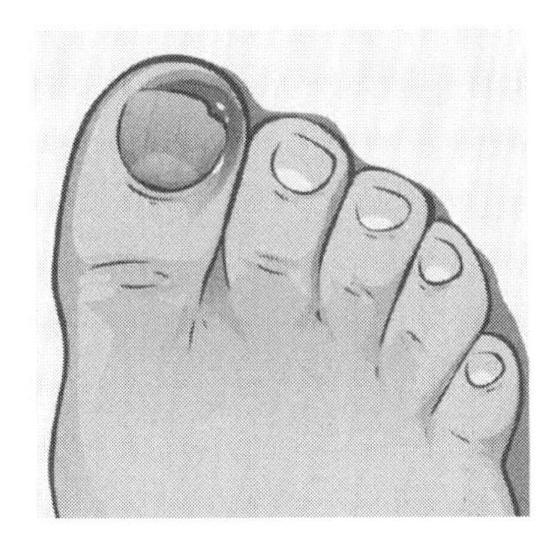

Naming the beast

Ingrown toe nail has several names. 'Ingrown' is the commonest and suggests part of its origin is growing into the flesh. If you are playing scrabble or want to impress others, you could say I have an onychocryptosis (on-ee-koh-kryp-toh-sis). IGTN is the shorthand version for ingrowing toe nail and used by health care professionals. The IGTN arises from three types of nail problem. Shape, break in the skin and bridging. In hands, we see a condition called 'Whitlow'. The skin on one or other side of the nail bed is inflamed and painful. A small amount of white discharge (pus) may be visible. Paronychia refers to the inflamed skin around the nail and is common to both toe and finger, so Whitlow just adds a name to provide further confusion. To appreciate the three toe types of IGTN, we need to know a bit of anatomy (p.166).

Can you die from an ingrown toenail?

Publicity and the nail are bedfellows, often for the wrong reasons. The blunt, if not misinformed, joke that someone is disabled infers that they shouldn't be through misconception of the magnitude of the condition. It is only an ingrowing toe nail, and therefore assumed minor. As a podiatrist, I have had an ingrowing toe nail, albeit mild compared to many of my patients, and the inconvenience and discomfort was far from amusing.

Whilst training, I was informed by my old Alma Mater[85] that you could die from an ingrowing toe nail. It appeared to stretch the truth by more than a mile. The only way you can die from an ingrowing nail is by spreading infection through cellulitis and septicaemia. Enter a real story from an Australian accident and emergency department. Such stories are rare but a 16 year old was reported in the Daily Mail.

I did of course apply some selective interpretation and appreciated that the newspaper wanted to get that wow – 'no-way headline!' but this was no fictional event. Sadly the teenager became sick and died after the clinical signs of danger had been ignored by doctors[86]. In another case in the UK, a young patient had her leg amputated after developing a rare pain syndrome following failed nail surgery.[87] This in fact is not so rare. Unlike the Australian case this was not negligent. I reported a case of complex regional pain syndrome in 1990 after nail surgery, but amputation did not follow and can confirm this pain syndrome is real but I can occur, although very rare.

---

[85] Literally means 'nourishing or fostering mother'

[86]https://www.abc.net.au/news/2019-09-09/alex-braes-death-still-haunts-doctors/11470424

[87]https://www.dailymail.co.uk/health/article-3819242/Teenager-ingrown-toenail-pays-5-000-leg-AMPUTATED-developing-agonising-condition-surgery.html

The moral of the tale is don't take an ingrown toenail lightly, or ignore infection.

Pain syndromes that cause dire decisions

Complex regional pain syndrome can occur after injury, infection or surgery and develop into the worst pain problem ever and this is what happened to the teenage amputee. Amputation is never recommended but fortunately in the case reported, it worked. The pictures on-line are VERY graphic.

Who are most at risk of surgical problems?

Those with poor immunity are at most risk and include patients treated with powerful drugs to suppress cancer cells. Immunity is about having sufficient specialist defence cells to ward off disease. Where patients have conditions such as leukaemia that impacts on the available quality of white blood cells, then great care is necessary with diseases and infection.

Does a 'V' cut help stop ingrowing nails?

This is a myth and old house wife's tale. It does not work. The nail grows from different parts of the toe and nail bed. While the front edge (hyponychium) contains some growing cells, you do not want to cut through this as it will bleed. The only way to stop a nail from growing is to destroy the nail growing cells. Don't let the previous story put you off if surgery is necessary. It is truly rare to die from an ingrowing nail but chronic infections lead to abscesses and misery and therefore should not be ignored.

Ingrown nail variations

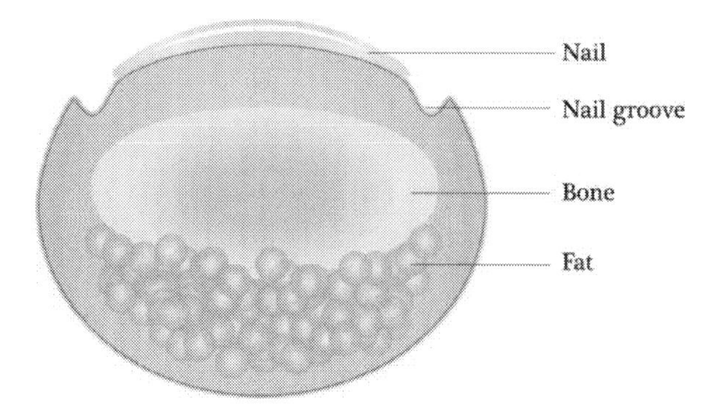

The hard nail is made from packed cells called keratin which sits on the softer part and at the end of the toe. It comprises a nail bed and two side grooves. The grooves form gutters that we call sulci (sulk-eye) or sulcus if singular. It is within the sulci that the problem occurs. The nail builds around a small area of inflammation. Let's deal with three scenarios.

Shape

The shape of nails varies widely in cross-section from flat to curved, as the edges of each nail sit in the sulcus. The more curved the nail at this point the greater the pressure against the skin where irritation can arise. The skin responds to pressure and thickens for protection. As the bulk of skin increases, it causes discomfort as it forms callus – thicker skin layers. Some nails are very curved (U.S.A– 'incurvated'), pinching off the skin. Sometimes only one side is affected. The incurved nail is the most common form and develops callus along the sulcus groove. The unique name – *onychophosis* is given to this hard skin. If you wonder about the terms used, anything starting with onycho- means nail.

Hard skin in the groove is not always painful, but given the right environment, such as a sporting activity where the great toe presses against a shoe, the nail squeezes against the groove and the underlying bone (phalanx). Pain arises with the inflammatory congestion —often erroneously called an ingrown toenail.

Break in skin

A true ingrown toe nail bears the name onychocryptosis. The nail edge penetrates the sulcus sufficiently to create two critical conditions. Initially, the skin is inflamed, and secondly, the wound created cannot heal and so overreacts, producing more healing material. This tissue is called hypergranulation.

As the skin attempts to heal, the repair process sets up a weak network of tiny vessels that, if disturbed, bleed. The colour is red and looks like a cherry on the side or end of the toe and requires professional help at an early opportunity.

Sweat makes matters worse and, of course, can cause that offensive smell which gives feet a lousy name.

The last ingredient that arises is infection. As long as the inflammation does not progress up the toe this can be managed with antiseptics.

The Bridge

The keratin from the skin attaches to the keratin of the nail. This can arise where the top surface of the nail separates slightly. Nails grow at a rate of 0.1mm a day[88] so you could expect slow tension placed where the bridge effect arises.

---

[88]https://www.healthline.com/health/beauty-skin-care/how-fast-do-nails-grow

As the nail moves forwards, the resistance of the bridging effect sets up a state of inflammation as it creates a drag effect. This condition can overlap with hard skin in the nail groove (onychophosis) but is more likely to start inflammation or callus build-up.

Avoid damaging the sulcus

Podiatrists do not recommend poking down the groove (sulcus). Maybe it is not as bad as poking around in the ear, but it is difficult to see what you are doing so far down the leg. As ear professionals have specially designed instruments that minimise damage, podiatrists use similar instruments. Adding local anaesthetic can ease discomfort and make inspection more thorough and pain free.

Do I have to suffer pain?

When it comes to treatment of the IGTN, you should not suffer pain. Modern foot care involves being offered a local anaesthetic as a standard if the problem is too painful to manage conservatively. You should not experience more pain than you would expect from a dental examination and treatment. If the clinician cannot provide this service, ask to see someone who can offer a local anaesthetic in an outpatient location. Only registered people trained as podiatrists or medically qualified people can provide local anaesthetics. If you are not provided with pain relief, and you feel you need it, then walk away.

Should antibiotics be used for the ingrown nail?

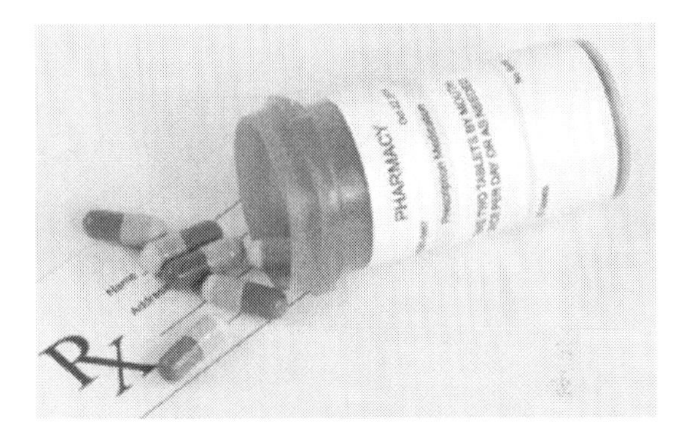

Antibiotics are not the correct treatment for an ingrown toe nail, although the infection will clear temporarily. Nail eruptions will continue until professionally managed. Antiseptics and good cleaning are imperative.

While patients should help themselves solve problems and prevent foot ailments, there is a narrow boundary between self-help and seeking professional help. Ingrown nails are not a condition to be managed without experience. At the first sign of inflammation, use a sterile plaster dressing and cover the skin and nail for 24-48 hours. If inflammation spreads or the toe swells, seek help.

When should antibiotics be used?

In truth, never. In reality, it depends if there is an actual infection and whether it has spread. Antiseptics still offer a place to help people offset against mild or early signs of infection.

If you are healthy and have uncontrolled diabetes or have immunological conditions, use antiseptics at the earliest opportunity. Any blood condition where the white blood cell count is lowered, as in leukaemias, may require antibiotics. Antiseptics will reduce the bacterial count lowering the risk of spread. A covering for a short time may soften hard skin to settle inflammation. If no improvement arises within 48 hours, then seek professional help.

Antibiotics will stop infection for a period. If a doctor gives you more than one course of antibiotic, then ask to see someone who specialises in managing ingrown toe nails. The reason antibiotics are not a fix is that the problem is based around mechanical irritation. If the spike or nail is not cleared the problem returns.

Dangers of overuse

Today more than ever, antibiotics must be reserved for severe infection and not heralded as a cure-all. Unless your infection spreads to your ankle or up your leg, then avoid this treatment. But, you can treat yourself for a short period with antiseptics and dressings. DO NOT use an A&E department. A&E departments are best for saving lives and stabilising serious medical problems, and this is where their primary skill lies. Other than this, junior doctors are happy to learn on your foot – is this what you want?

The worst ingrown nails include abscesses and an enlargement of the toe. I describe an occasion where a patient experienced an old fashioned approach to his IGTN in my book – *Podiatrist on a Mission*[89].

---

[89] [89] Tollafield D R Podiatrist on A Mission. The Dawning of a New Profession. 2021;41-2 & 48. Busypencilcase Communications. Amazon Books

Who should treat my nail?

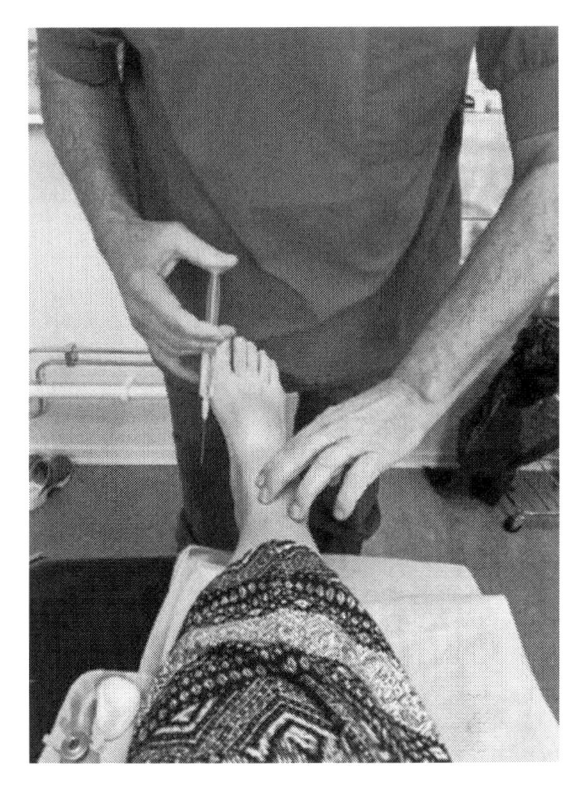

A modern outpatient setting where nail treatment can be offered in comfortable surroundings without having a full hospital admission is possible. Many patients prefer this to being admitted into hospital which today is less common than it once was. The clinician in the picture is feeling for the foot pulse but it should be noted that he is not wearing gloves!

Facts about phenol and gloves?

There is some evidence to suggest that gloves were originally used by the famous surgeon, Joseph Lister of antiseptic fame[90]. He used carboxylic acid as a spray and dressing. The chemical was damaging Caroline Hampton's hands as she acted as assistant to William Stewart Halstead, a US surgeon around the same time as Lister was active in the 1890's. Mercuric chloride was used as well as Lister's carboxylic acid. Gloves were therefore first used to protect the clinician and today this is still true. Any procedure that draws blood and can lead to infection is as much to protect the clinician as the patient.

HIV (AIDS) and hepatitis B made gloves mandatory in health care. However, and this is where there is a cross-over. Carboxylic acid is also known as phenol and used to treat ingrown toe nails. Phenol is so toxic to healthy skin a burn results. It was a curious observation but during the massive vaccination programme of 2021 in the UK, all the news clips represented injections given without gloves. Doubtless the savings in nitrile and rubber would have been significant.

Evidence & facts

An audit study comparing the medical and podiatry profession reported that podiatrists performed better than the medical profession for nail surgery results[91].

---

[90] Lindsey Fitzharris ISBN 978-0-141-98338-7. Penguin Books 2018 . First published in the USA by Scientific American / Farrar, Straus and Giroux. 2017

[91] Laxton, C. Clinical Audit of forefoot surgery performed by registered medical practitioners and podiatrists. J. of Public Health Medicine. 1995,17:311-315

Is it best to have a local anaesthetic or general anaesthetic?

There is no myth that an invasive procedure will hurt without pain relief. Much pain comes from the thought of a procedure based on anxiety. Patients are often keen to stay awake and have the type of pain relief offered by a local anaesthetic, much as we would at the dentist. Others would wish to be asleep, which entails a general anaesthetic. Modern medicine can deliver a middle road whether gas and air (nitrous oxide) as with child birth, or sedation given as a tablet or injection to calm us down. In this case there is no need for us to go to sleep. And so there is no straight answer – have what is best for you in discussion with your professional. BUT, there is no need to suffer pain.

Illness and risk

Doubtless for those at risk with certain medical conditions a general anaesthetic does come with inherent dangers and therefore it is best to remain conscious but comfortable. Once upon a time the death rate from surgery included anaesthetic mortality as much as death from infection. Modern surgery has made such leaps that most deaths today could either be avoided where they are called never-events[92] or an event arises which is not predictable. It might be erroneous to say with certainty that there are minor procedures, but there are certainly procedures which are more complex and risky.

[92] http://www.imperial-anaesthesia.org.uk/uploads/files/Never%20Events%20Analysis%20from%20London%20hospitals%20-%20final%20Imperial%20College.pdf

Anaesthetics and pain relief in podiatry

Here's a little known fact: between 1976-1985 all podiatrists in training schools learned the skill of local anaesthetics by practising voluntarily on each other. I wrote graphically about a true story in 1978. Two students injected each other and one fainted with colourful language.

"...In one corner of the clinic, Liz Farmer was being injected by another student, Deborah Brookes. A sudden shrill scream went up and she shouted, "You bloody fool... you've gone right through my toe!"

"I didn't mean to," Deborah apologised. "I couldn't help it... the needle is sharp!"

"Of course the needle is sharp. It's xxxx supposed to be!" Liz snapped, her voice carrying across the clinic.

Deborah, flush with panic, asked, "What do I do now?"

Fortunately, there were no patients, just senior students attending the course on local anaesthesia technique.

Dr Hamish Dalgleish, the consultant anaesthetist, soothed away these infractions in his calm Edinburgh accent. "Now come on, ladies. We need to be professional, there's no need for alarm. Just withdraw the needle."

<u>Current practice</u>

Podiatry students no longer practice on each other which in some ways is disappointing. Injecting into the skin of fruit is a substitute. However, there is no better way to broaden your knowledge than experiencing the same feeling and sensations as your patient.

6 - Footwear

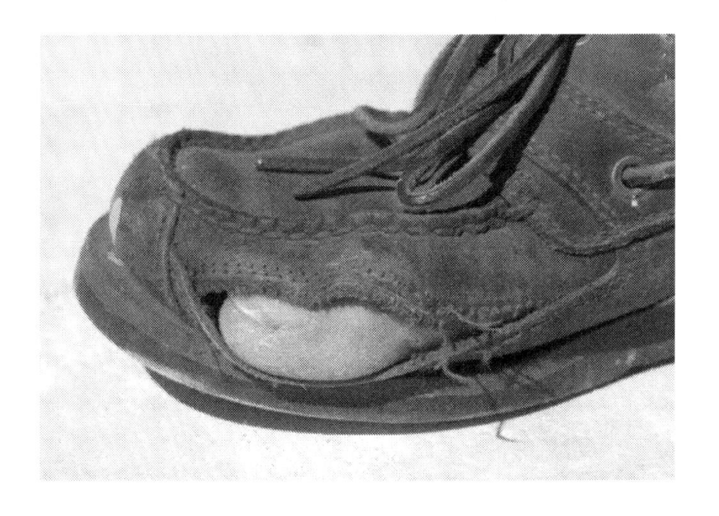

All podiatrists study footwear as part of their educational curriculum. Afterall, feet and footwear go together like a knife and fork. Sadly we wrestle with design and shape problems which fail to harmonise with all wearer's needs and can lead to avoidable foot health problems. The history of footwear is fascinating as is indeed the manufacture. There are shoe makers who make made-to-measure (bespoke) shoes, those that are concerned with the fashion of the day, and there are those dedicated products on the market that stand by their desire to offer quality shoes for children. Cheap and expensive can be found within the market place – on-line and on the high street.

This chapter does not cover the history of the shoe, but it does look a little at some of those esoteric aspects of footwear which might appeal.

- Wide shoes
- Narrow shoes
- Footwear markings
- Flat foot
- Measuring to fit
- Should high heels be banned?
- Myths from the grave.

Footwear and Martyrdom with feet

Fame and feet

The footballer David Beckham and his pop singer wife Victoria are brand names[93]. David inadvertently promoted the Aircast™ boot after experiencing a metatarsal fracture, while a tabloid newspaper photographed his wife with her bunions and shoes. Many shoes have developed for different purposes. Fashions often followed 18th century courtesans, but today pop stars and sports idols can make a difference by promoting fashion. Mrs B's foot shape did not look too bad, her shoes on the other hand were not sound for ideal foot health . Shoes have been regarded as the instigators of many problems. This is true but we need a bit of sympathy because those with deformity are disadvantaged. Unless a shoe can be handmade to fit (bespoke) then problems often arise due to pressure.

Wide shoes

The front shape of shoes are curious. The wider shoe shape is attributed to Henry VIII (1492-1547), the much revered and hated anti-papal English King, who wore wide shoes because of gout. Gout, as we covered earlier, is an inflammatory condition of joints caused by abnormal production of sodium urate associated with rich foods and a faulty metabolism.

---

[93] Sara Nathan 2009 Victoria Beckham shows off her pedicure (and bunion) as she loses a shoe
11 December 2009 http://www.dailymail.co.uk/tvshowbiz/article-1234900/Victoria-Beckham-shows-pedicure-bunion-loses-shoe.html#ixzz4HFlyi390

Given that Henry's high meat diet added to his weight gain and purulent legs in later life, one is not surprised he had foot problems and leg ulcers. Once the width of shoes impeded normal mobility, the trend eased back.

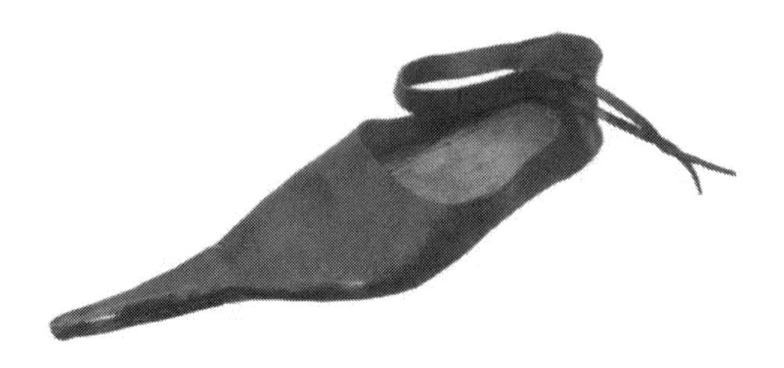

Narrow-pointed shoes

Shoes in medieval times were part of status. The medieval knight not only adopted long armoured shoes, but these were pointed. Long shoes were considered sinful and should only be worn by soldiers, according to the preacher Giovanni de Capestrano (1386-1456). This did not stop the fashion from spreading all over Europe[94].

During the period 1300-1500 the footwear style known as *Poulaines* became popular. While the origins seem to have emanated from Poland and named by the French, and possibly named from the ship's figurehead – polena, the shoe is reminiscent of those found in Middle Eastern footwear.

---

[94] Muzzarelli, MG In Shoes. A History from Sandals to Sneakers, ch.2 Sumptuous shoes. Ed. Blahnik, M. Published by Berg 2006:67-71

Footwear clues

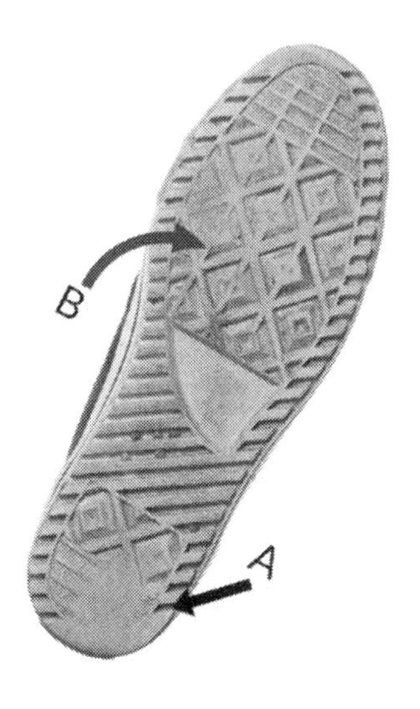

(A) Common to all shoes normal ground strike pattern
(B) Patterns under soles of shoes are easy give aways as they show wear more obviously when compared with patterns associated with less use.

Podiatrists can determine much from the state and condition of shoes. Pride and footwear go together. If shoes are comfortable we hang onto these friends for too long as the tread wears. Of course, the inner sole often deteriorates first and can damage the skin.

We should be familiar with normality. The sole depicted in the illustration above is not unusual where the lateral heel wear marks feature a foot that strikes the ground on the outside heel (A). However, the symmetry between feet should be equal in an ideal world. The type of patterns we see arise could be picked up by our forensic podiatrists, but also fall to all general podiatry practitioners. Excessive leg rotation, leg length discrepancy, rigid joint movements will all affect the foot. Then we come to conditions like the old 'flat foot'. The forefoot part of the sole should ideally be evenly worn down. (B) shows uneven wear. Design patterns that have unequal wear can show up walking styles influenced by muscles, tendons and joint function, as well as bone shape.

Flat foot

When it comes to treating flat feet, it is crucial to differentiate 'flexible' from the 'fixed' meaning, stiff foot. To work this out simply go on tip toe. If the arch height changes then you almost certainly have some flexibility. If the arch remains as before – suspect a stiffer foot.

The patient in constant pain needs investigating before using orthoses. Footwear should be evaluated and replaced. A shoe in one of my patients required replacing every six weeks, and the tread on the medial (inner) side showed excessive wear. As with car tyres abnormal tread raises an alarm that the steering may poorly aligned. And so the same exists with shoes and feet related to the lower limb linkage – *ankle bone connected to the leg bone*!

Frequent replacement with cheap shoes mean a shoe's life span is short and this sets up a cycle of continued shoewear and replacement. Purchasing footwear on such a cyclical basis is possibly more expensive than selecting a quality shoe to start with.

One must bear in mind that while medial wear is associated with flat feet, high arch feet can also increase medial wear. As the inverted (tilting outwards) heel moves inside the shoe, the heel counter (back) of the shoe gives way and breaks down. These changes are visible to anyone looking critically at shoes. It is a myth that only flat feet will cause inside wear on the heel. However one fact remains – we can tell as much about people from their shoes as could Sherlock Holmes.

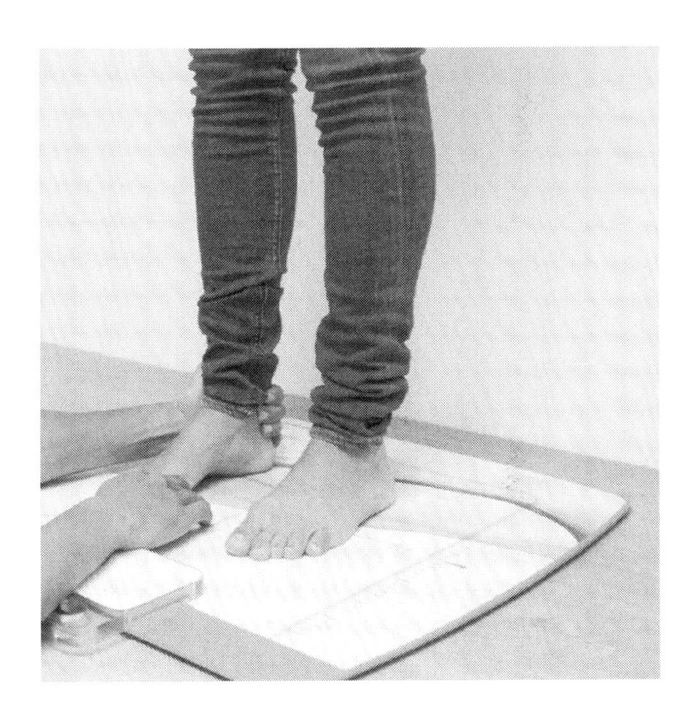

Should feet be measured when buying shoes?

In the UK in the fifties x-rays were used to assess feet for shoe fit in children. What a brilliant way to ensure toes were not scrunched up. Alas, x-rays give off harmful radiation. The giveaway is in its name. Today x-rays are regulated so that exposure to harmful radiation is regulated. One perhaps has to be older than me to recall such practices. I come from the age when a good shoe shop measured my feet with a metal or wooden slide and graduated lines to show shoe size. When I became an adult this all stopped.

Growing feet are easily harmed

True: Growing feet can be harmed by poor fitting shoes. Bound feet can take on a different shape. The story of the emperor's daughter or the Chinese Lotus dancer are anecdotal vestiges of a practice long gone. Feet do not have complete bones when we are born. An x-ray of a child's foot is interesting as there are gaps. The gaps are in fact not gaps but cartilage known as epiphyses. The epiphyses are the points where bone grows (p.69). Of course this is not just happening in feet. The clavicle or collar bone does not stop growing in males up to 25 years. Feet stop growing around 14-17 depending whether you are male or female. Males take longer to develop and are slower to mature – as we all know! The special cartilage in feet slowly turns to bone as we mature and becomes solid. Anything that distorts the cartilage will influence bone development. This makes children at risk even from poorly fitted socks, let alone shoes.

What are we measuring?

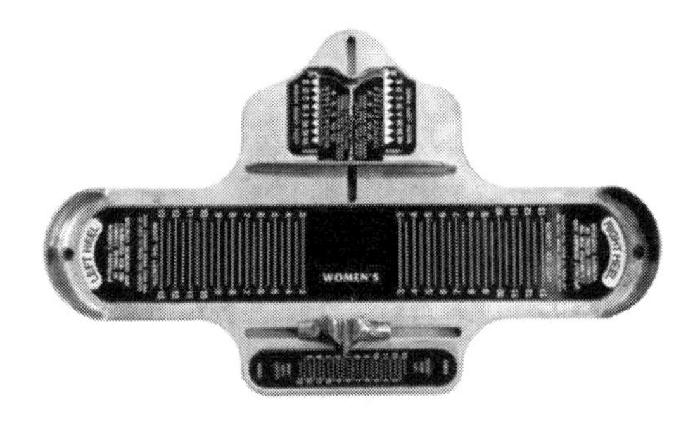

The length makes sense and ensures that we have a comfortable snug shoe. Length is given a size, but there are three conventional sizes. The British, the American and the European[95]. The British system started off as barley corns. Yes this is true, how many barleycorn grains made up the length of your foot. *Well, three barleycorns made an inch.*

Confusion arises because children and adults have different measures. When it comes to width we go to an alphabet so that narrow is A and wide is E. Then if you are very narrow you may have an AA or wider EE and so on. Width is not just how wide, but how fat your foot is across the top at its widest point. There are several conundrums here. Feet do not conform to one shape so at best you are using only two measures to achieve a best assessment of the size required. The foot can be so wide at the front and narrow at the back that gaps exist. Gaps mean rubbing. Rubbing means blisters, hard skin and pain!

---

95 https://goodcalculators.com/shoe-size-converter/

Nike ™, the sports footwear technology company made the following statement,

> "... a new scanning solution that uses a proprietary combination of computer vision, data science, machine learning, artificial intelligence and recommendation algorithms. It does this by measuring the full shape of both feet, offering the ability to know your truly perfect fit for each Nike shoe style. 2019"

All feet should be measured but bear in mind there are more parameters than just length and width. Furthermore, the circulation is made up of fluid being shifted by veins, arteries and lymph vessels. Some feet swell more than others. Pregnancy affects foot size where the foetus presses against large vessels impeding the efficiency of flow. Climates also affect feet size during the day and medical conditions like poor heart pumping and varicose veins have an effect on shoe size. Put together, the foot changes in size from morning to evening. For some, the only solution is to have two sizes in shoes to alternate between such changes. For the time being we must stick with barleycorns and a diversity of measurement, but make sure you know that an *American size* if different from a *British size*. Googling measurements and conversions (see footnote p.183) demonstrates the complexity.

Errors in shoe fit

Measurement is open to error and that error cannot be mitigated by two measurements alone. Trialling a shoe in a shop offers little guarantee when two days later that same shoe is found unsuitable. Take inlays along to ensure they fit. A shoe home trial was once acceptable from reputable family run shops. The industry has changed with on-line shopping.

But returns are possible from reputable companies; avoid making purchases where returns are disallowed.

Are high heeled shoes a new fashion?

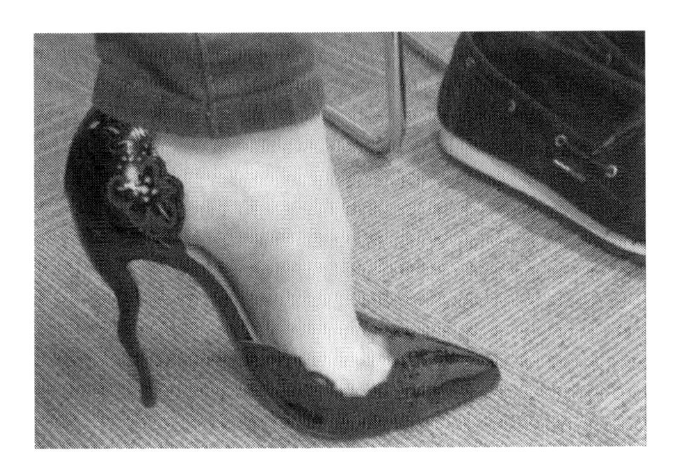

The Middle East was favoured as the source of the higher heeled shoe as with other patterns of design. High heels in Europe made their debut in the upper 16th century. Louis XIV gave way to this fashion which expanded to his male courtesans in particular. The shift in gender emerged as an exclusive feminine item by the early 18th century. Mary Wollstonecraft may have been one of the earliest critics that women used fashion to exploit their position represented in her book *A Vindication of the Rights of Women* (1792)[96].

---

[96] Semmelhack, E In Shoes. A History from Sandals to Sneakers, ch.11 A Delicate Balance. Women, Power and High heels. Ed. Blahnik, M. Published by Berg 2006:225-230

Should High Heels be Banned?

In this next section the myth about women's high heels continues and sources from modern newspapers help us consider the argument should high heels be banned?

> "The patient pulled out her new shoe with pride (illustrated p.185) and asked me what I thought? Her trainer can be seen on the other side of her left foot. The 42-year old had a significant hallux valgus on both feet and a bump over the midfoot."

Should the high heel be the bane of every podiatrist's life - *there are two views?*

For

The arch is elevated and can relieve some of the pain brought about by ankle tendon (tibialis posterior) contraction. The foot is often fully tilted (supinated), which does not need extra tendon pull.

Against

The heel cord tightens with excessive use and of course, lower shoe heights may not be as comfortable—the increased forces acting on the forefoot excites conditions like Morton's neuroma. A nipped off nerve between the 3-4th toes may be created and then scars and thickens as described earlier. The ball of the foot is exposed to shearing and frictional forces.

Small siliconised pads are used in shoes to reduce some of the pressure. Risks of injuries to the ankle and joints higher up the skeleton can arise. I looked for more information as to why women wear high heel shoes.

Are high heels and obsession?

In the USA, one survey identified the fact that 62 per cent of American women wore shoes with a 2-inch or greater heel regularly. The topic is discussed universally where fashion makes a powerful statement for both men and women. We find this is not entirely a female subject. But men's attitude to women has been challenged with some notable cases.

> "An RAF flight lieutenant who ruptured her Achilles tendon after being ordered to run with an 80lb kit bag in high heels has won her case for compensation at Preston crown court. Deborah Burns, now 28, was on the second day of her initial training course at RAF Cranwell, near Lincoln, in August 1996" [97]

Whose responsibility is it when it comes to using footwear? Nicola Thorp was 27 years of age when she made the headlines in 2017 in the UK. Her bosses at her Portico Agency required her to wear shoes from 2-4 inches high. A Portico spokesman said:

> "In line with industry-standard practice, we have personal appearance guidelines across many of our corporate locations. These policies ensure staff are dressed consistently and include recommendations for appropriate style of footwear for the role. We have taken on board the comments regarding footwear and will be reviewing our guidelines in consultation with our clients and team members. McDonnell, 2017" [98]

---

[97] The Guardian 20th March 2002. https://www.theguardian.com/uk/2002/mar/30/1

[98] RoSPA https://www.rospa.com/lets-talk-about/2017/january/high-heels-at-work

Flatgate

Journalists exposed the fact that not all women want to wear high heel shoes. McLaughlin, a journalist, reacted after the Cannes Festival where actors' flats' were barred from entry at the festival's red carpet event and called 'Flatgate'.[99]

British actress Emily Blunt was on the face of the media. A journalist told Blunt about the report that several women at Cannes were turned away from the red-carpet premiere of "Carol" because the festival mandates a high-heels-only policy when it comes to footwear. *"I think everyone should wear flats, to be honest,"* Blunt continued, *"We shouldn't wear high heels anymore. That's just my point of view. I prefer to wear Converse sneakers. That's very disappointing."*

Retaliation and rebuttal at the time of Nicola Thorp's event in 2017 ran in her favour from the Royal College of Podiatry (then called Society of Chiropodists & Podiatrists). The response was about safety at work and picked up by the Health and Safety executive (HSE), a government-backed body whose roots date back to 1833. That would put history at the time of the Great Reform Bill (1832), a political act, which changed the face of industry. The HSE published findings[100] but the UK Government rejected calls for a ban on enforced high heel wear. McDonnell says in her article;

> "What has not surfaced in the debate so far has been any real objective consideration of safety. Those employers who are keen to project a "glamour" image as part of their business profile also have duties to ensure, so far as is reasonably practicable, the safety, health and welfare of their staff.

[99] https://www.huffpost.com/entry/common-risks-of-high-heel_
[100] https://www.hse.gov.uk/slips/footprocure.htm

Slips and trips are a major cause of falls in the workplace and falls on the level, both at work and in public spaces, have been estimated to cost the UK £1billion annually."

Evidence of risk

Safety, above all, is a prime mover for ensuring that we all minimise accidents at work and, of course, at home. The problems with ankle damage naturally increase as the heel height elevates. Studies show that injuries due to wearing high heels (mainly sprains) have doubled over the past ten years – reported in an Alabama study[101.] Females, once considered shorter than men, might have desired more height, but in fact, this is not always the case, even though many tower over male partners. The effect of empowerment may have appealed to some possibly. For others, it allowed longer flowing dresses, maybe? It is just as likely some like high heels without any conditions. Hadley Freeman states;

> "(if) you understandably think women wear high heel shoes to be taller, [but] you are sorely underestimating the mental minefield that is to be a woman."[102]

> "Although high-heeled shoes might be stylish, from a health standpoint, it would be worthwhile for those interested in wearing high-heeled shoes to understand the risks and the potential harm that precarious activities in high-heeled shoes can cause."[103]

---

[101]https://www.sciencedaily.com/releases/2015/05/150521120924.htm
[102] https://www.theguardian.com/lifeandstyle/2015/jun/21/are-high-heels-bad-for-your-feet
[103] https://www.newsmax.com/Health/Health-News/high-heels-study-health/2015/05/22/id/646340/

Men's imposing attitudes on women sit poorly with today's view on equality. Nonetheless, it is a person's right to choose what they wish. And so, we need to seek evidence to find out more about the truth. Should those high heels be banned, and should podiatrists be keen to limit their use? And are there benefits to the higher heeled shoe?

Evidence of benefit

Cutmore, a podiatrist from New South Wales (Australia), advised health reporter for the Herald, Lisa Tait (1998) that while 10cm high heels made legs slimmer, the Achilles tendon could be destroyed slowly as the tendon shortened. Drawing some conclusion - before we ban any footwear, let us consider the benefits of high heels. While Cutmore knows that a shortened tendon makes walking difficult and causes foot pain problems in flat shoes, sometimes this is not always dependent on wearing high heels all of the time. Flat feet often do better with a heel height as it takes the strain off the inner tendons. While these are not as powerful as the Achilles, they are significant stabilisers of the foot. Moreover, plantar fasciitis occurs in regular shoes rather than high heels from my experience.

Facts

You need to use the proper footwear for the right job. Dress requirements need planning, weather conditions accounted for, and shoes should be selected for the type of walking surface encountered. Stilettos ideally should be interchanged when not required. If you choose to use these shoes, it is your right, but risks and the consequences of those risks could be long-lasting.

The myth from the grave

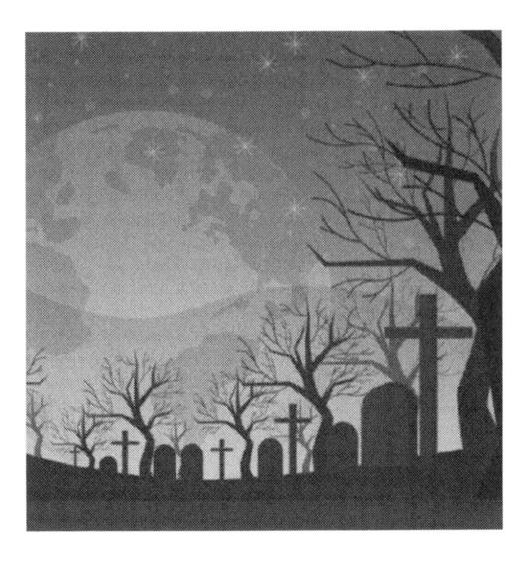

Following an excavation of bodies from sites around Ipswich, England,[104] a report was written tying footwear to the prevalence of hallux valgus. In fact, at the time of writing this book I found more references to archeological site excavations, but the Mays' 2005 report is sufficient for the point being made. Working from limited material, which often only allows visual bone damage around the first metatarsal, deductions were made about footwear and the deceased inhabitants from six centuries past. Mays concluded that the well-to-do were buried in parish grounds, because of access to wealth and therefore had a higher incidence of the deformity. The shoe type known as Poulaines, or the pike or spike type shoe, provided the cause. The assumption was based around the altered shape of the head of bone in the feet of the wealthy

[104] Mays, SA. Paleopathological Study of Hallux Valgus. American J. of Phys. Anthropology 2005;126:139-149

Dr Ana Deissler[105], a medieval footwear researcher makes shoes for sale and advises that there would be no way that Poulaines could cause hallux valgus as the leather is soft. The *myth from the grave* seems false despite the facts presented based on two grave sites; one with well-to-do people, the other site set away from consecrated ground. While May's report appeared as an attractive answer, it is flawed. Shoes do not cause deformity except in unusual circumstances. Restricting growth however will cause deformity as we saw when discussing the Chinese occupation with binding the foot and poorly fitted shoes and socks in immature feet. We learn that fashion often came from those at the top of the income pyramid and slowly filtered down in time.

The story of the human foot is still unfolding. The diversity that scientists have found in foot bones for australopiths[106] suggest there was variation in how they walked even among themselves. Archaeological excavations can still provide us with new information about the unique human and how we lived.

Isolated foot remains

Macabre though it seems, 21 isolated feet were found preserved in Canada in 2007 by a member of the public. No foul play was suspected but it was concluded that feet were often preserved in salt water. The footwear appeared modern (shown in the report)[107]. There have been reported incidents of feet being disposed following medical pranks without criminal actions!

---

[105] Deissler, Anna – author personal correspondence
[106] https://blogs.scientificamerican.com/anthropology-in-practice/what-makes-the-human-foot-unique/
[107] https://medium.com/internet-archaeology/the-macabre-case-of-the-21-severed-feet-of-the-salish-sea-71209d372a8e

7 – The Fable

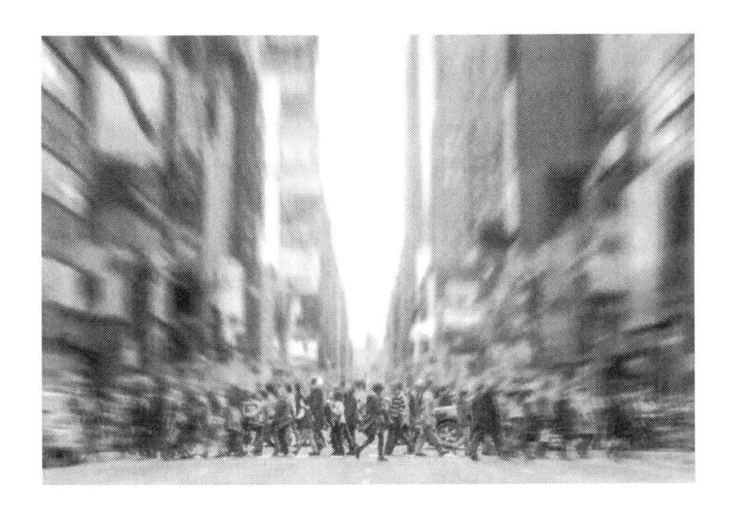

Don't you just love a good story. Some of the best come from Greek mythology and have found their way into novels and films. In this last chapter I look at myths, facts and science, where we can learn but must not be fooled. Unfortunately even scientists have been known to falsify their results, such are the pressures of university professors to publish a success story. And so we come back to ethics yet again. As a lover of Greek mythology I look at Androcles and Thetis.

- Follow the science
- The silicone experiment
- Moral of the tale

Myths, Fables and Science

Hopefully foot health myths are recognised only as ideas that have little credibility about treating problems. These stories, often known as old house wives tales, manifest over time and become legendary. Of course in some cases a bizarre treatment might work, but not for any scientific reason.

The use of dung to treat corns, recorded by Pliny the Elder, was cited in Dagnall's work[108],[109]. This may have been apocryphal as much as any past work written around the first century. But the use of soil and dung was recorded in early medical remedies and something the titans of medicine, such as Joseph Lister had to rebut, much to their own personal cost at the time. In the 18th century scientific evidence did not always stand up over prejudice. Contrast this with today and politicians trying to follow the advice of different groups of scientists with their so called 'Modelling Methods'.

Fables

Fables are somewhat different to myths although they contain fictitious stories but with that wonderful impact called the moral of the tale. To define a fable, a cryptic answer came from Gilbert Keith Chesterton, *"A fable can't be good with a human in it and a fairy tale can't be good without one.'* The best fables we learn come from many authors although Aesop is the best known. Others include Phaedrus, who may have in fact written fables attributed to Aesop, a humble slave. The Grimm Brothers, Rudyard Kippling, Guy Wetmore Carryl, Jean de la Fontaine and

[108] Colin Dagnall a podiatry historian of the 20th century. (1927-2015)
[109] Dagnall, J. A history of chiropody/podiatry and foot care. Br.J. Chiropody. 1983; 48:137-180

Joel Harris form just a small range of authors in a list of many. Hans Christian Anderson wrote a number of Fairy Tales and to some extent these were similar to fables. One could cynically have added that many myths about feet are just Fairy Tales! The one described is attributed to Aesop who remains the father of the fable and concerns the foot. Animal and human come together.

Androcles[110]

"A slave named Androcles once escaped from his master and fled to the forest. As he was wandering about there he came upon a lion lying down moaning and groaning. At first he turned to flee, but finding that the lion did not pursue him, he turned back and went up to him. As he came near, the lion put out his paw, which was swollen and bleeding, and Androcles found that a huge thorn had got into it and was causing all the pain. He pulled the thorn and bound the paw of the lion, who was soon able to rise and lick the hand of Androcles like a dog. Then the lion took Androcles to his cave, and every day used to bring him meat from which to live. But shortly afterwards both Androcles and the lion were captured, and the slave was sentenced to be thrown to the lion, after the latter had been kept without food for several days.

The emperor and all his court came to see the spectacle, and Androcles was led into the middle of the arena. Soon the lion was let loose from his den, and rushed bounding towards his victim. But as soon as he came near to Androcles he recognised his friend, and fawned upon him, and licked his hands like a friendly dog. The emperor, surprised at this, summoned Androcles to him, who told him the while story. Whereupon the slave was pardoned and freed, and the lion let loose to his native forest."

---

[110] https://owlcation.com/humanities/fables-

MORAL: Gratitude is the sign of noble souls.

Lions and humans

The Androcles fable is curious because we see the Thorn Boy, a statue with a thorn reflecting pain. The Bible has stories about 'Daniel in the Lions' Den' where divine intervention saves Daniel from certain death. Samson slew the lion with his strength as did Hercules, the latter completing the first labour when taking on the Nemean lion. All these protagonists failed to examine the lion's foot in each case but Androcles. Maybe these feet should be left to a vet!

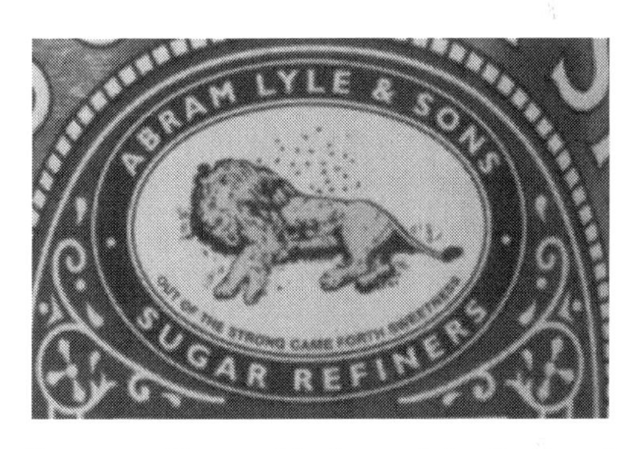

Manufacturers, Tate and Lyle used the lion attributed to Samson on their product.

"Lyle had strong religious beliefs, which is why the tin's famous logo depicts strongman Samson's 'lion and bees' from the Bible's Old Testament, registered as Lyle's trademark. 'Out of the strong came forth sweetness', as the quote goes; where bees produce honey inside the lion's carcass, rich syrup pours from the well-loved tin... And the logo and design remain unchanged to this day (along with the delicious contents, of course)."

Again we see advertising associated with fables tied to a story depicting a biblical figure. Clearly fables have both human stories and stories associating animal characters with human characteristics. We should reflect on past teachings and try to make something of how myths have crept into science. I suppose it is a little like Chinese Whispers so loved of those birthday party experiences. Messages inevitably become distorted. While this book covers myths and facts in the main, there is one moral to the tale that contributes to modern interpretation of foot fables.

"Beware of false promises on a book's cover for the content may deceive and deliver disappointment." Author

Achilles

There are few who won't know the part of the ankle called the achilles tendon and many might know the myth that someways gives rise to a fable about our immortality.

When Achilles was born, Achilles' mother, Thetis tried to make him immortal by dipping him in the river Styx. However, she held him by the left heel. Greek mythology is complex and Achilles is invincible until when attacking Troy (now Turkey). He takes an arrow in his heel and dies. Tragedy was loved by the Greeks. However bringing this powerful and important tendon away from mythology we learn that the tendon has a poor blood supply and when damaged can produce problems. A case of a 60 year old man who loved gardening developed infected cellulitis from a small crack in his achilles tendon. Modern medicine saved him and his leg but it required a skin graft and surgery to clean the wound. The moral to the tale is that we cannot assume injury without consequences and even gardens are dangerous places because of micro-organisms found in the soil. Perish the thought that Pliny the Elder thought dung would make a useful dressing.

Getting the wrong end of the stick!

I wrote a book called *"Morton's Neuroma. Podiatrist Turned Patient: My Own Journey"*. The key point was that the title reflected the content as the story was of ME the patient as much as THE clinician-author. I read a ONE STAR Amazon review. This came from a Canadian reviewer –

"Doctor seems to spend more time talking about himself than helping anyone else." It occurred to me that the reader, to whom I am truly grateful, may have misread the title of the book!

Some of those kind enough to read *this* book may say, *I want more about self-help*, and indeed why not. This is a self-help book in one way but not a do-it-yourself book because the point about myths and facts is simply that.

It is important to look at common foot conditions so that everyone can determine their origins. Of course I am keen to ensure people do find solutions to their foot problems but as one reviewer constantly says to me, *the foot is a complex structure*.

Be careful what you read and do not believe all promises made. When writing my book on bunions (published in 2019) I saw other books with a similar title that started with; '*how to cure..*' and '*how to fix a bunion without surgery*'. Past books are only mentioned as part of my duty as an author and clinician is to provide factual evidence of value. Books can be misleading and the content often ambiguous. Those with a high price tag, with few pages, offering a naff cover, and written with little expertise, disappoint.

Finding more self-help and foot health

You can use my website consultingfootpain.co.uk where I provide self-help and factual information, or you can look out for books on foot disorders and reviews. The resources are building, based on a project I started in 2014 when writing for patients. I wanted people to have the benefit of helping themselves before seeking professional help. This was not an altruistic philosophy. Patients who could sort their own problems needed broad advice first. If successful, pressure could be removed from the NHS and GP practices. When consulting patients I hoped that all elements of primary care had been covered which would make my own work easier. Like blowing away cobwebs, the corner of the room becomes clearer and easier to organise than if left. When talking to those with foot problems it is easier to know if basic methods have been used first e.g antiseptics for a wound.

For the most part many readers will use a Google or Bing search which are still the most popular while Yahoo, Ask and AOL are lower down in the top 10. Finding facts has never been easier, but the downside is having to wade through the plethora of adverts.

There are text books that may appeal, but these are aimed at students of podiatry and professionals as they contain complex descriptions and require background knowledge.

Closing subjects

In the last two sections, I will – *'Follow the science'* – that often quoted statement by politicians. For the reader, a sizable moral sits behind the last tale – *The Silicone Experiment.*

Following the science

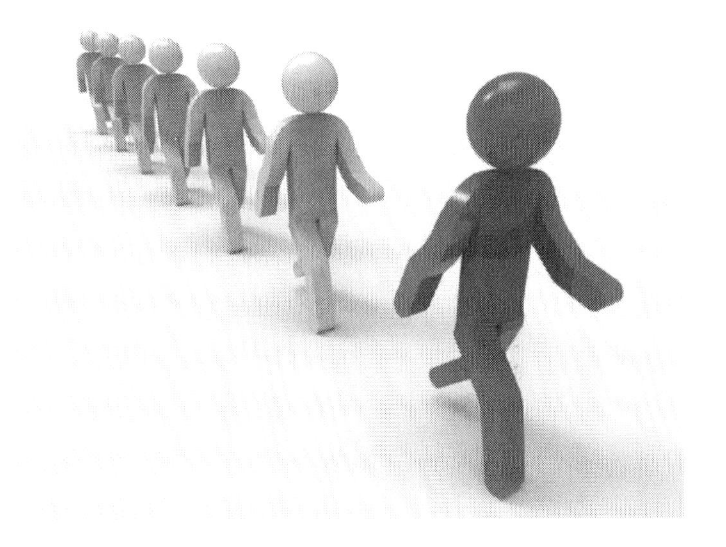

A cautionary tale

'Follow the science' has become popularised during the Covid-19 years and forms the basis for decision making using evidence. Many ancient brews worked because some of the ingredients had medicinal benefits, but the doses could be hit and miss. Other concoctions served as little more than placebos. No-one sets out to harm people unless there is criminal intent in mind or psychiatric instability and belief. Harold Shipman (GP) is possibly the worst person who killed patients between 1995-1998, while Ian Paterson (breast surgeon) maimed his patients through acts of greed and hubris.

Science will reduce the risk if experiments are carried out conscientiously, but we have to go further and always test all medicines and products against existing medicines or against something that is harmless, like water or coloured candy. Yes, I am aware that colours are dyes and such ingredients themselves can cause allergies – this highlights the problem. On one occasion my colleague shouted out – *'have you seen the list of instructions in their warning sheet for this injectable?'* The substance was sterile water!

Advertising

Advertising is a different dimension and offers promise and benefit from products either tested to a high standard or follows a basic premise that they work for some. It is a tricky subject because to sell goods, like a politician trying to sell a policy to an unyielding public, one has to sugar coat the benefits. Abram Lyle's Golden Syrup benefitted from a little poetic licence, but some manufacturer's go further. In the foot health market, one distributor advertises ingrown toenail paint. Now you would not want to put this on an infected nail and clear guidance should be observed within the product information. As with all medicines sometimes this can be overwhelming and puts fear into the user.

Advertising by the distributor hoping to recoup any investment can overtake the ethical undertones whereby a product is deemed reliable.

Good experimental design

We must call one group *a control* to avoid bias and those who perform drug trials must remain unaware of the source of the volunteers, which means the control being used, or the active ingredient being unknown. This makes the trial *'blind'*. It is a little like playing battle ships. Until the end you do not know whether your missiles are on target or not.

Evidence based medicine

The subject of science and evidenced based medicine would fill several books but the best myths come from skin products. The advert may say tested on a certain percentage of people and then you realise the percentage value of 90% relates to only a few. The problem is worse. The numbers a product is tested on, called the population-N may not be representative of the population at all and could be biased.

Take a survey of friends who share your views. How reliable would it be if you relied on their responses for your results to be equated to the general population. Larger numbers drive down error, but to make a valid statement about reliability, the numbers must be large enough to help us decide if that product, medicine or device, is helpful.

We can take this further and say we must study only a certain age group, those who are healthy and without known disease and reactions. We may find products that are designed for certain groups be they female, male, from an ethnic group or gender variation.

For some, medical science has learned, to its cost, that many treatments are not suitable for some groups, and if there has been any benefit from the pandemic in 2019-21, we have learned how some groups of people are more sensitive and at risk than other groups.

I will leave you with a trial never recorded before - one which podiatry colleagues and I ran in 1996. Myths, facts and fables collide in this tale – *The Silicone Experiment.*

The silicone experiment

The work of Dr Sol Balkin[111] has passed into podiatric history for two reasons. Firstly, because the method he applied worked for him, but secondly, when tested under strict scientific conditions the method failed. It is a tale that is hidden from the public and to some extent few will know of the case.

Balkin was an American podiatrist from Glendale, California, and spent most of his career developing a method to replace lost fat in the foot. It was his aim to cure corns and callus. In this respect all podiatrists yearned for that magic cure. Doubtless, Balkin (1915-1994[112]), benefitted many patients. His ideas were of concern because of the unknown effects of silicone within the lymphatic system as well as uptake of unwanted particles in the liver.

A Company called Biodermis (US), supported Balkin to launch the product in the UK but required the manufacture of the medical grade silicone to be approved under the European Union in Eire. The work was conducted at a podiatry centre in the Midlands, UK with full ethical approval and later published in a scientific journal in 2001[113].

---

[111] Balkin, SW Plantar keratoses: treatment by injectable liquid silicone. Report of an eight-year experience. Clin Orthop Relat Res. 1972 Sep;87:235-47.

[112] The citation of Balkin's death is probably inaccurate as the author did not start work with Balkin until 1995-6.

[113] Tollafield DR, Holdcroft DJ, Singh R, Haque MS. Injectable Percutaneous Polydimethicone in the Treatment of Pedal Keratomas: A Single Blind Randomized Trial. Foot and Ankle Surgery. 2001. 40(5):295-301

Scientific analysis

Having been informed that a medical grade silicone could cure corns under the ball of the foot based on longstanding work by Balkin (1972), a trial using two groups was set up to record results. This has the name PROSPECTIVE as opposed to retrospective, where this type of study reviews older data accepting flaws in study design which cannot be controlled.

A control group – (A - water) and an active group (B - medical grade silicone) were introduced and the two products were randomly allocated to reduce bias so the volunteer patient did not know whether they would receive dose A or B. After several injections the volunteers were followed up and photographs shown to an independent scrutineer. The volunteers all returned their final opinion based on pain experienced and how they felt about their treatment and if the corn had been cured.

Random biopsies were taken to consider the effect of silicone and ensure no active inflammatory changes arose. Biopsies were conducted by punching a 3mm piece of skin from the area, which is a little like taking a sample of water to see if it is contaminated. The results showed water was no more or less effective using an agreed dose of injected silicone. The trial successfully demonstrated the limits of silicone for corns on the sole of the foot.

Two further findings arose

Where silicone was injected in toes, the results were much better, but the numbers studied were too low to be reliable. It is likely, had more funding, time and subjects been made available, Balkin's original work may have gained acceptance within the medical community.

Moral of the tale

Ten years on, two of the volunteers required surgical removal of the silicone from their feet because the ingredients caused deep tissue reaction. Fifteen years on a further patient required the silicone removing. And, so we learn - following the science has many aspects.

It can teach us much if the experiment known as a trial is performed ethically and to a high standard.

The second most important aspect relates to following volunteers for long enough after trials because in the final analysis we have to look at the risks as an unwanted byproduct. In the case of dermal silicone injections for corns, the benefits could have been huge and the profits from developing this high.

Epitaph

Sadly Balkin died with deep disappointment that his personal project, one that had taken him many years of development, suffered from an outcome that he had not predicted. It took courage to try to help patients and there was nothing mischievous or intentionally wrong or even unethical. All Balkin's patients consented, but the level and degree of consent in the 21st century is at a very high ceiling today. The UK trial was undertaken with Balkin's full permission and he demonstrated his technique to us. Balkin's original success required large volumes of silicone to work on the sole and offered impressive photographic results originally. However, he had never subjected his work to the rigours of a scientifically controlled medical trial until the UK study. If an experiment cannot be repeated faithfully by an independent observer then the method or science must be questioned.

One does not need to be medically trained or have vast scientific knowledge to appreciate how the Corona virus vaccination process has been rolled out to millions, with concerns over small numbers of fatality. Humans place a high store on safety and this is unlikely to diminish.

Medical care of the foot

In 2019 Professor Cathy Bowen, one of the clinical leads based at the University of Southampton engaged in a project covering referral patterns. This was supported by the Musculoskeletal Alliance. Only 3% of patients presenting to GPs had encounters relating to foot and ankle pain. This represented 567,000 in real numbers. Diabetes has the highest awareness rate but arthritis as an entity enjoys less recognition. During 2019-2021 the effect on health care services is likely to have an adverse impact as the foot is at risk of falling below the radar in terms of keeping our population active and independent. This remains the top priority for the podiatrist.

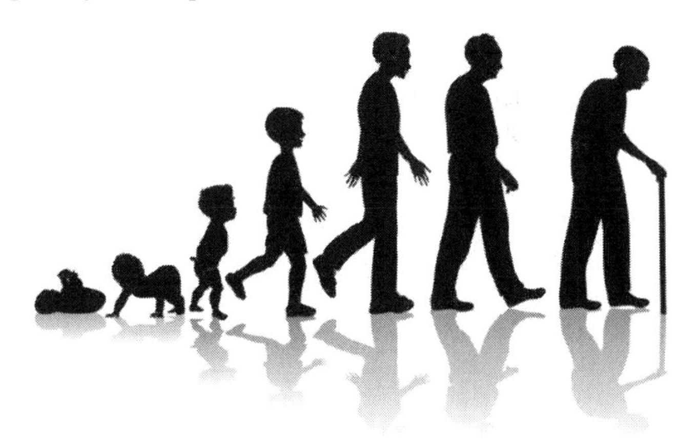

About the author

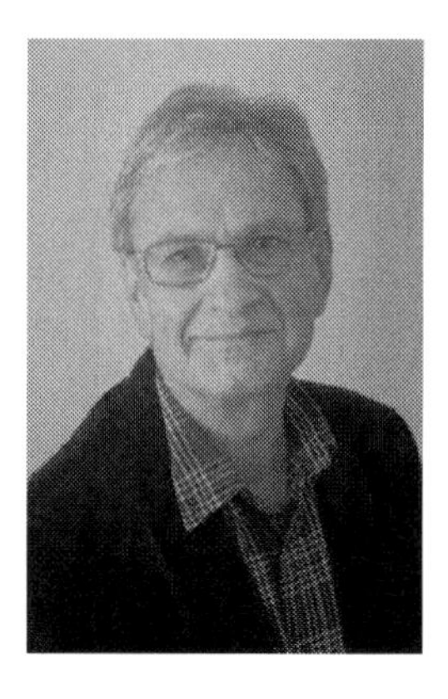

David is passionate about podiatry and believes in the importance of promoting foot health and knowledge through case illustrations and encouraging people to take up podiatry as a career. He is a former consultant podiatric surgeon, clinical researcher, educationalist and is still registered. He has worked for both the education and NHS sectors as well as latterly joining an Independent hospital. Although retired, he is a Fellow of the Royal College of Podiatry and an Affiliate member of the University of Huddersfield. As a full-time writer-author and public speaker he lives with his wife in the West Country and divides his time between writing and amateur dramatics, Nordic walking, travelling and researching medical and military history. During 2021 he produced several new titles, one, a short fictional book *'Fatal Contracts'* available from Amazon. He has also written a children's book for his grandchildren (published in 2014 – private sale only through his site).

Acknowledgements

While this book is undoubtedly my creation and therefore any mistakes and views are mine alone, I would like to credit the physiotherapy department at Spire Little Aston Hospital for inviting me to talk on the subject of feet in 2016. In putting the presentation together, a number of conditions emerged revealing some of these myths and facts.

My second inspiration came from Israeli podiatrist, Caroline Semah, who trained in the UK and was kind enough to invite me to speak in Tel Aviv. It was here that the myths, facts and fables really started to take shape amongst a mixed group of professionals - podiatrists, orthopaedic surgeons and dermatologists. I have built on these with time and what was a small book has grown after my manuscript lay dormant. It has given me great pleasure to produce this book and show appreciation to colleagues who have supported me.

To Dr Grace Parfitt of the University of Huddersfield who assisted me with their excellent library and references. Reaching out for evidence is an important requirement for any non-fiction author so we do not make things up! To Professor Wesley Vernon, OBE, a specialist in forensic podiatry who added his story and Daley Denning who has impressed me with his thoughts behind our fitness centre at LED. My cover designer Petya Tsankova, patient as always in supporting me and improving my production mistakes. To my beta readers, Sid Gibson, Shaun Global, Jane Clare and latterly Professor Tim Kilmartin for writing the foreword to this book. Last but not least, to my wife, Jill, who guides me with a touch a ruthless criticism but keeps me on the right track. I am truly grateful to her for the careful, watchful and cautious eye she brings to my writing.

A personal word

Thanks for reading this book which I hope provides a useful insight into foothealth or even sets you on the road to our wonderful profession of podiatry. All authors, especially ones who are independent and self-publish, rely on word of mouth and recommendations, and so any genuine feedback, if you feel that you can spare the time, would be appreciated.

A number of references used in this book have come from my own resource centre and are on my website consultingfootpain, if not available on open-access.

To communicate please use busypencilcasecfp@gmail.com and I will reply personally

---

You can sign-up to my free newsfeed located on my website landing page. Other books covering foot health are available from Amazon and listed in the front of this book. Please follow me on Facebook @david.tollafield or LinkedIn or Twitter @myfootjourneys.

David R Tollafield
FRCPodS

Index

X

Learn more about Podiatry

Podiatrist On a Mission. The Genesis of a New Profession.
David R Tollafield. 2021.

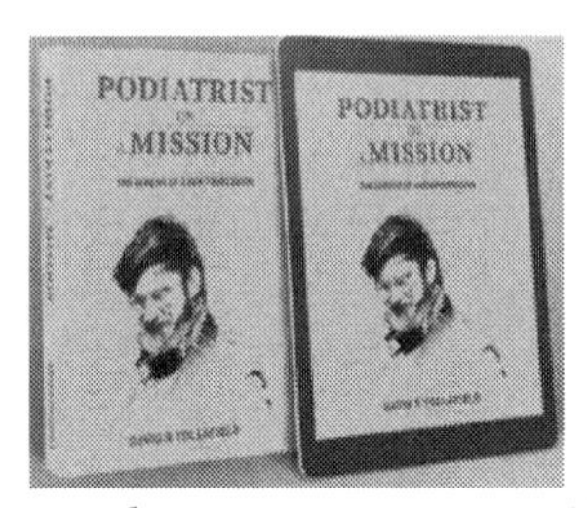

Read an extract on page 174
Available from Amazon books (e-book and paperback).

If you enjoyed this introduction to the world of foot health and podiatry why not read about when podiatry emerged from the older profession of podiatry in this autobiographical novel by the same author. From failed A levels to professional, from chiropodist to podiatrist, podiatrist to lecturer, lecturer to foot surgeon.

This "intrepid frontiersman" emerges with others as heroic pioneers forging a new future. The story concludes just as we want to know more and what becomes of this author and his mission. *Professor Alan Borthwick*

It is a fantastic story, riveting. I read it for pleasure and what a pleasure it was. You have managed to create the atmosphere of the early years so well. *Professor Tim Kilmartin*

For me, it was a page turner... brilliant. *Alison Charlton*

As a novel I simply loved reading your story...it is a book to remind us of how far podiatry has come and the obstacles you had to negotiate to get us here. *Janet McGroggan*

Easy to read and enjoyed it immensely. *Rob Hardie*

Printed in Great Britain
by Amazon